The Fit Back

Prevention and Repair

Fitness, Health & Nutrition was created by Rebus, Inc. and published by Time-Life Books.

REBUS, INC.

Publisher: RODNEY FRIEDMAN
Editorial Director: CHARLES L. MEE JR.

Editor: THOMAS DICKEY
Executive Editor: SUSAN BRONSON
Senior Editor: MARY CROWLEY
Associate Editors: WILLIAM DUNNETT, CARL LOWE
Chief of Research: CARNEY W. MIMMS III
Assistant Editor: PENELOPE CLARK
Copy Editor: LINDA EPSTEIN
Contributing Editor: JACQUELINE DAMIAN

Art Director: JUDITH HENRY
Associate Art Director: FRANCINE KASS
Designer: SARA BOWMAN
Still Life and Food Photographer: STEVEN MAYS
Exercise Photographer: ANDREW ECCLES
Photo Stylist: LINDSAY DIMEO
Photo Assistant: TIMOTHY JEFFS

Test Kitchen Director: GRACE YOUNG
Recipe Editor: BONNIE J. SLOTNICK
Contributing Editor: MARYA DALRYMPLE

Time-Life Books Inc. is a wholly owned subsidiary of

TIME INCORPORATED

Founder: HENRY R. LUCE 1898-1967

Editor-in-Chief: JASON MCMANUS
Chairman and Chief Executive Officer: J. RICHARD MUNRO
President and Chief Operating Officer: N.J. NICHOLAS JR.
Corporate Editor: RAY CAVE
Executive Vice President, Books: KELSO F. SUTTON
Vice President, Books: GEORGE ARTANDI

TIME-LIFE BOOKS INC.

Editor: GEORGE CONSTABLE

Executive Editor: ELLEN PHILLIPS
Director of Design: LOUIS KLEIN
Director of Editorial Resources: PHYLLIS K. WISE
Editorial Board: RUSSELL B. ADAMS JR., DALE M. BROWN, ROBERTA CONLAN, THOMAS H. FLAHERTY, LEE HASSIG, DONIA ANN STEELE, ROSALIND STUBENBERG, HENRY WOODHEAD
Director of Photography and Research: JOHN CONRAD WEISER
Assistant Director of Editorial Resources: ELISE RITTER GIBSON

President: CHRISTOPHER T. LINEN
Chief Operating Officer: JOHN M. FAHEY JR.
Senior Vice Presidents: ROBERT M. DESENA, JAMES L. MERCER, PAUL R. STEWART
Vice Presidents: STEPHEN L. BAIR, RALPH J. CUOMO, NEAL GOFF, STEPHEN L. GOLDSTEIN, JUANITA T. JAMES, HALLETT JOHNSON III, CAROL KAPLAN, SUSAN J. MARUYAMA, ROBERT H. SMITH, JOSEPH J. WARD
Director of Production Services: ROBERT J. PASSANTINO

FITNESS, HEALTH & NUTRITION

The Fit Back
Prevention and Repair

Time-Life Books, Alexandria, Virginia

AAV 4096

CONSULTANTS FOR THIS BOOK

Deborah Caplan, a Registered Physical Therapist, specializes in back care and the Alexander Technique. A founding member of the American Center for the Alexander Technique, she is on the senior faculty of its teacher training program. She is the author of *Back Trouble: A New Approach to Prevention and Recovery Based on the Alexander Technique.*

Michael G. Neuwirth, M.D., an orthopedic surgeon, is Chief of Scoliosis Service at the Orthopedic Institute of the Hospital for Joint Diseases in New York. He is also Assistant Clinical Professor of Orthopedics at Mount Sinai School of Medicine in New York.

Luanne Sforza, a Registered Physical Therapist, is Director of Physical Therapy at the Sports Training Institute in New York City, where she specializes in the rehabilitation of musculoskeletal and sports-related injuries. She developed the institute's Healthy Back Program, which she administers.

Elaine Stillerman is a licensed massage therapist and vice president of the Alliance of Massage Therapists, Inc. She is an instructor at the Swedish Institute of Massage in New York City.

Judith C. Trobe, a Registered Physical Therapist, is a back specialist in private practice in New York. A former faculty member in the physical therapy departments at both the University of Pennsylvania and the University of Florida at Gainesville, she has been a corporate consultant on preventive back care to General Electric. She is a certified instructor of the Alexander Technique and frequently lectures on back care.

Nutritional Consultants

Ann Grandjean, Ed.D., is Associate Director of the Swanson Center for Nutrition, Omaha, Neb.; chief nutrition consultant to the U.S. Olympic Committee; and an instructor in the Sports Medicine Program, Orthopedic Surgery Department, University of Nebraska Medical Center.

Myron Winick, M.D., is the R.R. Williams Professor of Nutrition, Professor of Pediatrics, Director of the Institute of Human Nutrition, and Director of the Center for Nutrition, Genetics and Human Development at Columbia University College of Physicians and Surgeons. He has served on the Food and Nutrition Board of the National Academy of Sciences and is the author of many books, including *Your Personalized Health Profile.*

For information about any Time-Life book please call 1-800-621-7026, or write:
Reader Information
Time-Life Customer Service
P.O. Box C-32068
Richmond, Virginia 23261-2068

First printing.
Published simultaneously in Canada.
School and library distribution by Silver Burdett Company, Morristown, New Jersey.

TIME-LIFE is a trademark of Time Incorporated U.S.A.

Library of Congress Cataloging-in-Publication Data
The Fit back: prevention and recovery. — 1st ed.
p. cm. — (Fitness, health, and nutrition)
Includes index.
ISBN 0-8094-6114-5.
ISBN 0-8094-6115-3 (lib. bdg.)
1. Backache—Popular works. 2. Backache—Prevention. 3. Back—Protection.
I. Time-Life Books. II. Series.
RD771.B217F57 1988
617'.56—dc19   88-12374
                                 CIP

This book is not intended as a substitute for the advice of a physician. Readers who have or suspect they may have specific medical problems should consult a physician or certified therapist about any suggestions made in this book. Readers beginning a program of strenuous physical exercise are also urged to consult a physician.

CONTENTS

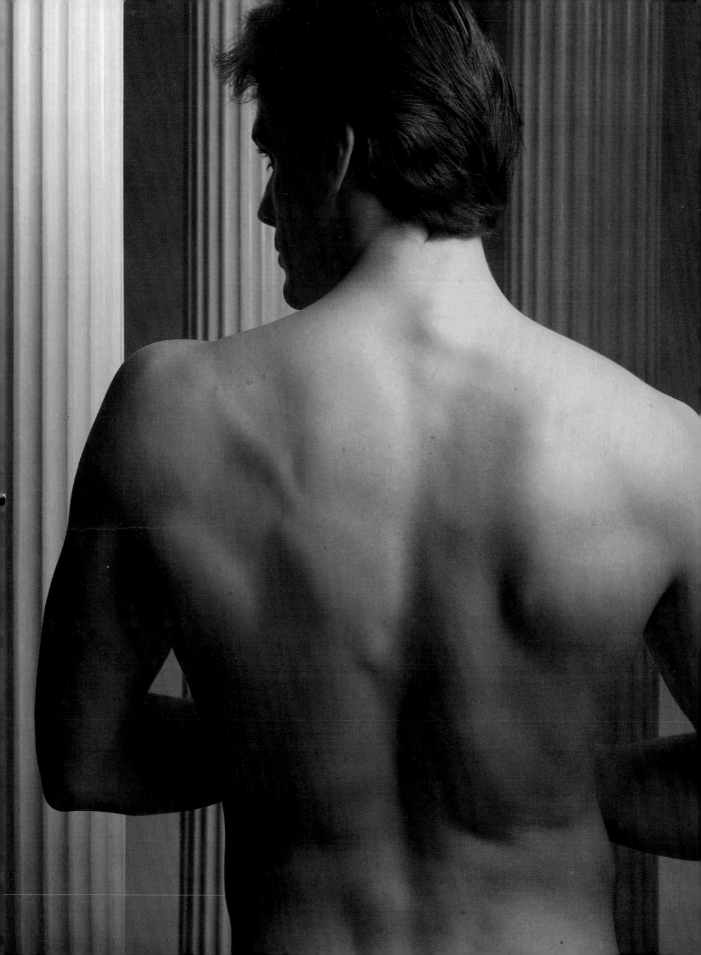

CHAPTER ONE

How Your Back Works

Its strengths and weaknesses, why backs ache and the dramatic benefits of exercise

A fit back is strong and resilient, capable of absorbing a multitude of shocks every day and of supporting loads far greater than your body weight. In well-trained athletes, a single disc in the lower back has been shown to bear loads in excess of 2,500 pounds. Yet eight out of 10 people, including those who are generally fit, experience some type of back pain during their lives. Back problems rank second only to the common cold as the most frequent cause of sick leave in the United States, and Americans spend an estimated five billion dollars a year to treat their backs.

Much of this suffering and expense is avoidable. The great majority of backaches stem from muscular problems that can be prevented or alleviated with improvements in posture and exercise and other lifestyle habits. Indeed, exercising regularly is the most important step you can take to protect your back. This chapter explains back mechanics and guides you toward effective ways to ease a troubled back or keep a fit back at its best.

Why should you be concerned about your back?

Just as a bad back can interfere with everyday activities, a fit back can assist you in leading an active and healthy life. The human spine — extending from the base of the skull to the tip of the tailbone — is one of the most complex and vital parts of the body. Rather than a single long bone, the spine consists of an intricate network of interlocking bones called vertebrae, fluid-filled cushioning discs, connecting ligaments, important nerves, and numerous small and large muscles that support the back (see illustration opposite). This unique structure is integrally involved in almost every movement you make, from picking up the phone to walking.

Although the spine is designed to accommodate everyday movement as well as the demands of exercise, it has potential weaknesses that age and repeated patterns of misuse — inactivity, poor posture habits, improper lifting, sitting in badly designed chairs — can accentuate. If your back is weak, a movement as minor as a sneeze can trigger back muscle spasms. It is therefore prudent to care for your back before problems arise.

What causes back pain?

To some degree, all back trouble stems from degeneration. As you age, the cushioning discs separating the vertebrae of your back begin to lose their elasticity and moisture, and they shrink. This can lead to a variety of conditions ranging from simple muscle pain to more damaging problems such as a herniated disc. Although more than 100 causes of back pain have been identified, the majority of cases are the result of injured muscles and ligaments. One large-scale university study found that 83 percent of backaches could be attributed to weak or tense muscles.

Contrary to popular belief, backs do not just "give out." An accumulation of problems, including wear and tear on insufficiently toned muscles, poor posture, obesity and stress, are predisposing factors. A simple move, such as bending to pick up groceries, can aggravate already weakened muscles, and it may lead to a protective but painful mechanism: The muscles in the back go into spasm — sustained involuntary muscular contractions — to guard you from further damage. By immobilizing the back, the spasm forces you to take the best course of action and lie down. This position not only places the least amount of stress on your back, but it allows inflamed tissue to repair itself.

Back pain varies in intensity from nagging to excruciating. The degree of pain is sometimes a good indication of the type of injury or illness, but sometimes it is misleading. Certain diseases and serious illnesses can produce low levels of back pain, while muscle spasms, which usually clear up within days, can trigger agonizing pain.

If back pain is accompanied by any change in bowel or bladder habits, decreased sexual function or numbness in the genital area, you should contact your physician immediately. These symptoms can

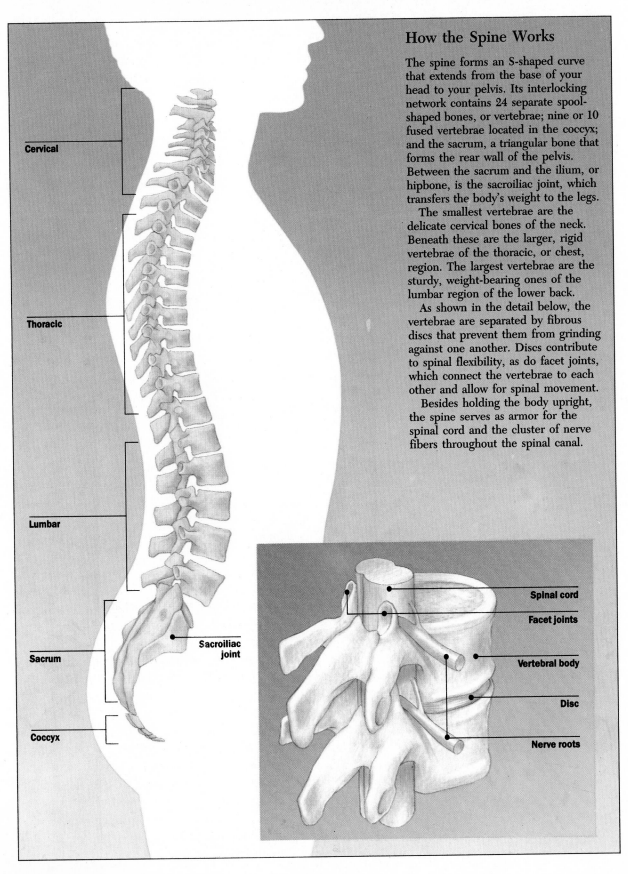

Cervical

Thoracic

Lumbar

Sacrum

Coccyx

Sacroiliac
joint

How the Spine Works

The spine forms an S-shaped curve that extends from the base of your head to your pelvis. Its interlocking network contains 24 separate spool-shaped bones, or vertebrae; nine or 10 fused vertebrae located in the coccyx; and the sacrum, a triangular bone that forms the rear wall of the pelvis. Between the sacrum and the ilium, or hipbone, is the sacroiliac joint, which transfers the body's weight to the legs.

The smallest vertebrae are the delicate cervical bones of the neck. Beneath these are the larger, rigid vertebrae of the thoracic, or chest, region. The largest vertebrae are the sturdy, weight-bearing ones of the lumbar region of the lower back.

As shown in the detail below, the vertebrae are separated by fibrous discs that prevent them from grinding against one another. Discs contribute to spinal flexibility, as do facet joints, which connect the vertebrae to each other and allow for spinal movement.

Besides holding the body upright, the spine serves as armor for the spinal cord and the cluster of nerve fibers throughout the spinal canal.

Spinal cord

Facet joints

Vertebral body

Disc

Nerve roots

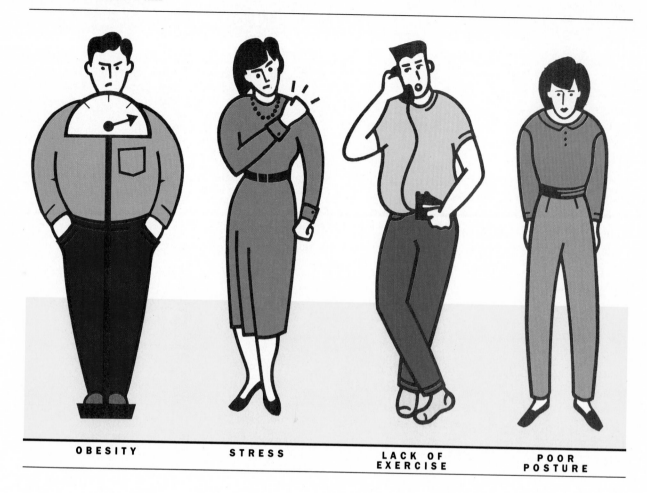

| OBESITY | STRESS | LACK OF EXERCISE | POOR POSTURE |

Each of the four factors illustrated above contributes to the likelihood of your suffering back pain. Both obesity and poor posture throw the back out of alignment, straining muscles and ligaments. Stress, the factor over which you may have the least control, can contribute to muscle tension, which increases the risk of injury and can lead to muscle spasm. A sedentary lifestyle is doubly troublesome: Weak muscles fail to support the spine properly, and too much sitting causes muscular strain.

indicate a nerve disorder that necessitates emergency surgery. Back pain accompanied by vomiting or fever or any back pain in a child should get prompt medical attention. Also, any back pain, numbness or tingling that radiates down your arm or leg, while not an emergency, should be evaluated immediately. Otherwise, experts agree that a physician need not be contacted unless pain persists after two or three days of bed rest and aspirin or another analgesic.

Who suffers from back pain?

Although back pain can affect anyone, it is more likely to occur if you are between the ages of 30 and 55. The average age of patients who undergo lumbar-disc surgery is 42. Because older women are more prone to osteoporosis, the bone-weakening disease, they face greater risks than older men.

Backaches afflict workers at all levels in all occupations, and those with the least physically demanding jobs may be just as vulnerable as those whose jobs are strenuous. A recent 10-year study at an Eastman

Kodak plant found that nearly half of those who performed heavy physical labor sought treatment for lower back pain and nearly as many sedentary employees also sought such treatment. Sedentary white-collar workers suffer back pain because they spend long hours sitting, often in poorly designed chairs; many blue-collar and service workers can blame their back trouble on repeated and improper lifting and carrying.

Why do most backaches occur in the lower back region?
The largest curve in the back is formed by the five vertebrae of the lower spine, which comprise the lumbar region. These vertebrae, the largest in the spine, support the most weight and are also subject to the greatest strain from such activities as lifting, bending and twisting. These factors make the area much more vulnerable to injury than the relatively inflexible thoracic spine in the middle back and the cervical spine in the neck, which, although more mobile, does not bear as much weight as the lumbar spine.

Can back pain signal other health problems?
Fully 80 to 85 percent of back pain is muscular in origin, and another 5 to 10 percent is due to a bulging or ruptured disc. Other back pain may signify an underlying disease or a structural problem. In these cases, back pain can be a symptom of scoliosis, an abnormal sideways curvature of the spine, arthritis or, in rare instances, infections or tumors. Also, backache can signal trouble elsewhere in the body. Kidney and heart disease, as well as prostate, uterine, ovarian, pancreatic and liver problems, may all have back pain as a symptom.

How does poor posture contribute to back problems?
Many experts believe that improper posture places too much stress on the spine. When correctly aligned, the spine curves gently inward at the neck and lower back, and outward in the rib area. This modified S shape keeps the head, chest and pelvis centered over one another, balancing the weight of the body. Compromising this posture with rounded shoulders, a slumped sitting position or an excessive arch in the lower back creates weight imbalances that put added strain on the back. Over time, such strain narrows the spaces between the vertebrae. In certain cases, the result is a bulging disc (see illustration, page 13). Fortunately, posture is an area that can be improved dramatically. To evaluate your posture, see pages 22-23. A series of exercises that will help you improve your posture is shown in Chapter Three.

Do sports and other fitness activities help the back?
In general, activity is good for the back. Not only does exercise improve back support, but recent research demonstrates that it directly benefits the discs. A study by an internationally renowned back expert in Sweden showed that exercise aided the flow of nutrients to spinal

discs, possibly delaying their deterioration. Indeed, the only way that discs can receive nutrients is through movement.

Regular exercise is essential for back strength and flexibility; studies have shown that even cardiovascular exercise can improve back problems. However, most popular forms of exercise do little to help strengthen muscles that support the back. Too often exercises can exert uneven pressure on the back, tightening and straining the muscles as a result. Although there are numerous cases of professional athletes sidelined by back trouble, most back pain afflicts the novice or weekend athlete, and research has proved that unconditioned exercisers who push far beyond their limits are more likely to injure their backs than are everyday fitness enthusiasts.

If you exercise regularly without back trouble, there is no reason to discontinue doing so. However, you will benefit by adding back-strengthening exercises to your fitness regimen, and making sure to warm up sufficiently before a workout. If you are subject to back problems, you should avoid certain sports and activities likely to aggravate your condition, specifically those that involve lifting, twisting, arching the spine, sudden starts and stops, and falls or collisions. One survey found that 25 percent of golf pros suffer from lower back injuries caused by the exertion of twisting. With care, you can modify some of the twisting activities in the sports that encourage back trouble *(see box, page 97)*. Harder to adapt are sports like football and basketball. One study found that football linemen had among the highest incidence of lower back pain among athletes.

Is it true that simply walking upright is the main reason humans have so many back problems?
This is a common misconception that is based on neither evolutionary nor anatomical fact. Indeed, the spine is a marvel of evolution that allowed human beings to walk upright, thereby freeing their hands for more productive use. And walking on four legs is no assurance of a trouble-free back; certain breeds of dogs develop herniated discs. Also, degenerative arthritis of the spine has been found in birds and reptiles, among other species.

Is sitting all day a major cause of back pain?
Spending too much time sitting in a chair can certainly exacerbate back trouble, especially if your sitting posture is improper. A famous Swedish study found that sitting exerted 75 pounds more pressure on the lower back of a 150-pound person than standing did *(see illustration, pages 14 -15)*. Slumping does not support the lower back, and hunching your shoulders tenses the neck and upper back muscles. However, sitting properly in well-designed chairs can help.

What other activities create back problems?
Any activity, if performed improperly and done repetitively, can weaken the back. Particular offenders are lifting and bending in ways

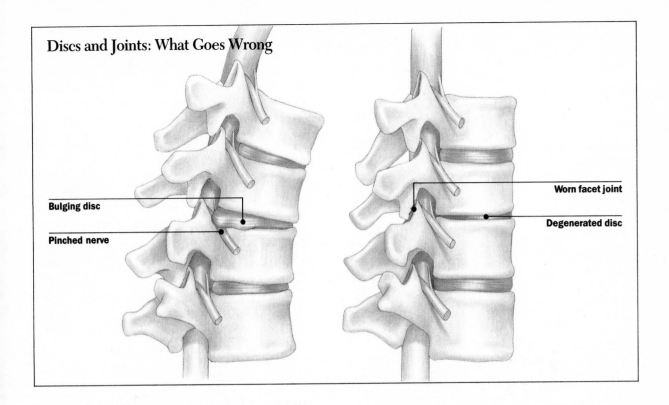

Discs and Joints: What Goes Wrong

Bulging disc

Pinched nerve

Worn facet joint

Degenerated disc

that greatly exaggerate demands on the spine. Comparing lifting with bent knees and lifting with straight knees, the Swedish study noted on page 12 found that the improper straight-leg lift places an additional 285 pounds of stress on the spine. Proper lifting and bending techniques, as well as suggestions for easing strain on the back caused by daily activities, are shown on pages 100-115.

Can backaches be triggered by stress?

Stress can certainly make you vulnerable to back trouble. One recent study of pain and its relationship to stress found that 46 percent of Americans reported feelings of stress at least once a week; 35 percent experienced it less than once a week; and 16 percent said they never experienced stress. Those with high levels of stress are much more likely to experience all kinds of pain than those with low levels. Sixty-nine percent of the high-stress group reported backaches in the previous year, as compared with 49 percent of the group that reported feeling stress once a week or never. One of the physical manifestations of stress is a chronic shortening and tightening of muscles, and many researchers claim that psychological stress can actually trigger muscle spasms. Such back muscle problems can overstretch ligaments and place excess strain on the spine, making it much more prone to injury. Keeping your back muscles flexible with the exercises on pages 56-67 will help alleviate this stress reaction.

Most back pain is muscular in origin, but structural problems with discs and joints are sometimes responsible. Disc problems occur when pressure from surrounding vertebrae causes a disc to bulge *(above left)* or even rupture. Such deformities can impinge on a nerve, producing intense, radiating pain. As a person ages, discs degenerate, causing them to lose moisture and become thinner. This allows the facet joints to rub against one another *(above right)*, wearing away their protective coating and causing painful problems such as osteoarthritis. A worn facet joint can also rub directly against nerves and cause pain.

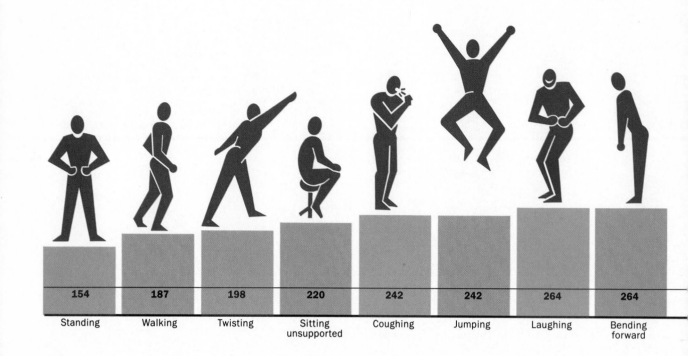

| 154 | 187 | 198 | 220 | 242 | 242 | 264 | 264 |
| Standing | Walking | Twisting | Sitting unsupported | Coughing | Jumping | Laughing | Bending forward |

How similar are neck pain and lower back pain?

Except for the fact that it is less common and less likely to cause total disability, neck pain is essentially the same as lower back pain. Unfortunately, neck pain, which more often results from a traumatic injury like whiplash than from misuse, is not as responsive to exercise treatment as lower back pain is.

Will your back be helped by a specially designed chair or a firmer mattress?

The positions in which you sit and sleep are much more important than what you sit or sleep on. Because everyone's body is different — height, weight, leg length, spinal curvature — sitting and sleeping needs are also individual. Finding the proper chair or mattress for you may take some experimentation. No matter what type of chair you choose, try to find those that you can modify to suit your own back. A well-designed chair adjusts to your height and can accommodate your back needs. If you sleep comfortably on your current mattress, keep it; if you do not, first try to improve your sleeping posture, as shown on pages 118-119. Otherwise, you should consider buying a different mattress or using a bedboard.

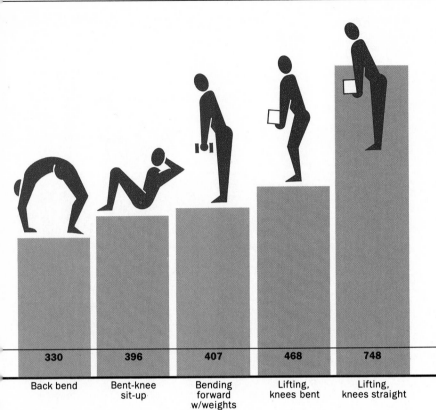

330	396	407	468	748	**Pressure on Lower Back (pounds)**
Back bend	Bent-knee sit-up	Bending forward w/weights	Lifting, knees bent	Lifting, knees straight	

A Swedish study comparing the amounts of stress the back sustains from various activities turned up some unexpected results, as this chart shows. A good belly laugh and coughing place more stress on the lower back than either walking or twisting. Lying down (not illustrated) was the least stressful activity, with just 66 pounds of pressure for a 150-pound adult. The worst activity was lifting an object without bending at the knees, which created 748 pounds of pressure. The measurements were based on readouts from an electronic gauge implanted in the third lumbar vertebra of a healthy woman.

Does diet have anything to do with your back?

Although back pain strikes the average-weight as well as the overweight person, there is some evidence that excess weight, particularly in the abdomen, can contribute to back trouble. A potbelly creates the same problem as weak abdominal muscles: Both throw off the body's center of gravity by pulling the lumbar spine forward into an excessive curve, thus compressing the vertebrae. By maintaining your ideal weight, you will eliminate one contributing factor to back pain. For more information on the connection between your back and your weight, as well as lowfat recipes to help in weight maintenance or reduction, turn to Chapter Five.

What can you do when back pain strikes?

The traditional prescription for backache used to be one to two weeks of bed rest, but recent studies have shown that two days is sufficient, on average. This shortened period of bed rest also gives muscles less time to atrophy, which can further complicate back problems. After you rest and the pain has subsided, stretch your back gently to relieve pressure on the nerves. If severe pain persists after you have spent two days in bed, you should contact your physician.

Fit Body, Fit Back

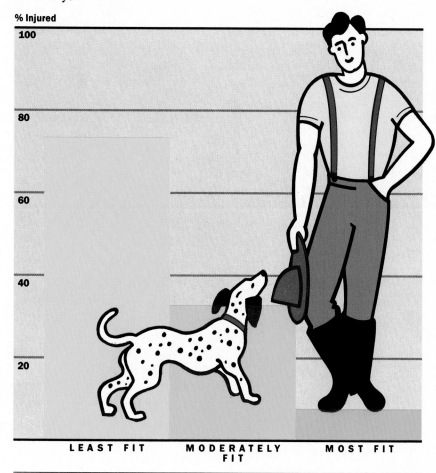

% Injured

A study of 1,652 firefighters underscores the importance of fitness for a pain-free back. Based on tests of their cardiovascular endurance, muscular strength and flexibility, the firefighters were divided into three groups: most fit, moderately fit and least fit. Researchers traced their back injuries for three years. Back problems were virtually nonexistent among the most fit, while almost 80 percent of the least fit firefighters suffered injuries.

LEAST FIT   MODERATELY FIT   MOST FIT

In conjunction with bed rest, you can take analgesics, such as aspirin or ibuprofen, to reduce both pain and inflammation. In addition, most experts agree that heat is soothing to muscles in spasm; you should apply it repeatedly for 15- to 20-minute intervals. Although back-care professionals disagree on the value of icing an injured back, the general tendency is to use ice if it seems to help, especially immediately following an injury that affects a local area of the back. Wrapped ice packs should be applied for 10 to 20 minutes every two hours for the first two days.

What is a slipped disc?

In fact, it is a misnomer, because there is no such thing as a "slipped" disc. Discs are firmly anchored between vertebrae, and, while they may be subject to considerable degeneration that can create serious problems, they cannot become dislodged. Composed of strong yet flexible fibrous tissue filled with a gelatinous center, discs serve an important role in the spine: By separating the vertebrae, they allow the spine to bend and curve, acting as a shock absorber.

What is often referred to as a slipped disc is actually a disc that has partially collapsed or ruptured as a result of degeneration and strain. When a disc ruptures, or herniates, the outer tissue of the disc tears, allowing the softer material to ooze into the spinal canal. This can lead to severe pain if the disc material presses on a nerve. A bulging, preruptured disc can cause the same sort of pain. However, if the disc never presses on a nerve, you might not even be aware of the condition. *(See illustration, page 13.)* Such a rupture is usually the mechanism behind sciatica, a very painful condition caused by pressure on the sciatic nerve, which runs along the back of the hip and outer side of the leg.

Fortunately, such disc problems account for only 5 to 10 percent of all back trouble. And of this percentage, only a small minority require surgery. Up to 90 percent of those with disc problems respond to the traditional, conservative treatment for back pain: bed rest, analgesics, heat and perhaps physical therapy. In these cases, rest allows the disc to heal itself by reducing inflammation and reabsorbing the extruded material responsible for the pain.

How long does it take for back pain to subside?
Most back pain subsides within 10 days to three weeks, although the outer limits of this recovery period extend to three months. Only 5 percent of lower back pain patients have symptoms that persist for more than three months, and even with the more debilitating sciatica, 50 percent of patients recover within a month.

What is the best way to prevent back trouble?
Studies show that those who are the least physically fit are more likely to have an acute lower back injury. The current consensus among experts is that strengthening and stretching the back with exercises that focus on the back-supporting muscles and, equally important, retraining those muscles to move so as to place the least strain on the back, are the best ways to ensure a healthy back. In addition to its preventive value, regular exercise can diminish chronic pain. Chapter Two of this volume presents back-strengthening exercise routines that match your fitness level.

By keeping your muscles and joints in correct equilibrium, good posture goes hand in hand with strengthening your back. Combining posture and strength to facilitate good back movement day to day is shown in Chapter Four.

It is sometimes possible to avert a bout of back pain if you rest as soon as your back feels fatigued, then gently stretch the back muscles. The Back Attack routine on pages 26-29 is designed to relax muscles by stretching tense muscles and ligaments.

How to Design Your Own Program

Many people accept back trouble as an inevitable nuisance, but they are doubly mistaken. A bad back is not inevitable, but often is related to your lifestyle or to habits that heighten your vulnerability. And if a backache that starts out as just a nuisance is ignored or attended to only intermittently, it can suddenly become very painful.

The questions at right will help you assess whether you are at particular risk for lower back pain. After you answer them, take the simple tests on pages 20-23, which will measure the condition of the muscle groups that offer the most protection against back problems.

Are you a candidate for back trouble?

1 How old are you?

Although back problems can strike adults of virtually any age, the most likely victims are between 30 and 55. During this age span, the spine's discs — which are composed of cartilage and fluid — lose some of their inner moisture and shrink, a phenomenon that partly explains why you may become slightly shorter after you reach middle age. As this degenerative process occurs, either the vertebrae themselves or the facet joints that connect vertebrae to each other may rub together, and such friction is a common cause of backache. After the age of about 55, though, the disc degeneration ceases and the spine assumes a more permanent and rigid configuration that makes it less prone to back disorders, with the exception of osteoarthritis.

2 Have you ever had back pain?

Someone who has had even one episode of back pain is at greater risk than someone who has never experienced such pain: Your chances of having a recurrence within two years are about 3 to 2. Unless you have a structural problem in the spine, which can cause recurring back pain, the subsequent episodes can probably be traced to your lifestyle and body mechanics, which include the way you stand, move or lift objects. If your standing and movement patterns strain the muscles in your lower back, you must first become conscious of your bad habits and then try to correct them. You may be able to head off future attacks by practicing good posture, exercising and utilizing other strategies shown in the three following chapters.

3 Are you overweight?

Nearly everyone would like to lose a few pounds for appearances' sake. But if you are obese — that is, if you weigh more than 20 pounds above the ideal weight for a person of your height and build, the excess pounds may strain your back by creating a gravitational pull on the muscles that support it, especially when the extra weight is carried in the abdomen. Also, overweight people are more likely to be out of shape than their leaner counterparts, and muscle weakness is strongly associated with back problems. A sensible weight-loss program, combined with muscle-strengthening exercises, will help.

How is your posture?

...yback posture that exaggerates the normal lumbar, or lower back,
...ve can be troublesome. Overarching strains the muscles and ligaments
...his area, placing undue pressure on the lumbar vertebrae. Contrary to
...e outdated notions, proper posture does not require a rigidly straight
...e, but rather an alignment that follows the spine's natural curves.

Are you under a lot of stress?

...e precise role that psychological stress plays in causing back problems
...ains elusive, but many researchers believe that because it creates mus-
...tension, stress alone can trigger a back attack in some people. If your
...ss level prevents you from relaxing, muscular tension can occur
...oughout the body, and particularly in the neck, shoulders and back.
...relieved tension strains these muscles and decreases their mobility,
...ich may lead to back pain. Research has shown that an exercise program
...n effective stress reliever. A back massage, such as that shown on pages
...-123, can also provide relief.

Do you do housework or yard work?

...nding over and pushing a vacuum cleaner, lifting a toddler or straining
...reach a high shelf are the occupational hazards of homemakers. Such
...ivities can be just as stressful to the back as heavy labor. A day of rak-
... leaves or gardening can be as hard on the back muscles of an unfit
...son as several sets of tennis are to a weekend athlete. Shoveling snow,
...ich requires bending, lifting a heavy load and twisting the torso, can
...o pose serious hazards. Both at home and elsewhere, proper lifting and
...nding techniques, demonstrated on pages 104-105 and 110-111, can go a
...g way toward sparing your back.

What kinds of exercise do you do?

...scles need exercise to stay toned and firm; for back care, the muscles of
... back, abdomen and thighs should get special attention. The best pre-
...iption is for a regular, moderate endurance-exercise program that gives
...u an aerobic workout three times a week for 20 minutes or more, com-
...ed with the special back-care exercises in Chapter Two.

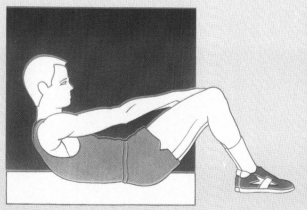

Abdominals/1: Lie with your knees bent. Tilt your pelvis back to flatten your lower back. With your arms outstretched, lift your shoulders and upper back. If you cannot hold this position for at least 30 seconds, your abdominal strength is poor.

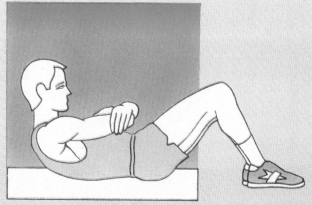

Abdominals/2: Start in the same position as for the previous exercise, but this time cross your arms over your chest. Lift your upper back off the floor and hold. If you can maintain this position for at least 30 seconds, your abdominal strength is fair.

How Strong Is Your Back?

As with any fitness program, the best approach to conditioning your back is progressive: If your back-supporting muscles are weak, they must be strengthened gradually. While the basic back exercises in this volume are gentle enough for almost anyone without acute back pain, the advanced routines are designed for those who are quite fit. Do not attempt the more rigorous exercises before you have built up adequate muscular strength. Overzealousness at any point during an exercise program can sideline you.

The exercises on these two pages evaluate the strength of the muscles that are most important for supporting your back — your abdominals, back extensors and quadriceps. Based on the amount of time you can sustain each exercise, you will be able to rate your back strength as poor, fair, good or excellent. The four sit-up variations above test your abdominals progressively; if you can do the first, advance to the second, third or fourth. Evaluate your quadriceps strength with the wall slide at right, and test the strength of your back extensors with the back lift at far right.

The results of these strength tests will steer you to the most suitable exercises in Chapter Two: If you are in the poor category, start with the basic routine on pages 40-45. If your rating is fair, turn to the moderate strengtheners on pages 46-51. And if your muscle strength rates either good or excellent, you can try the advanced routine on pages 52-55.

If you fall into more than one category — say you are good on the abdominals test but poor on the back-extensor test — choose the easier routine instead of combining basic and intermediate exercises. It is important to let your weaker muscles catch up, thereby developing a full support system for your back.

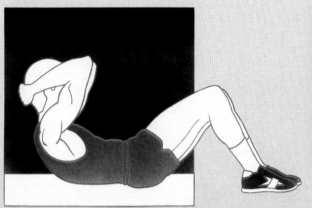

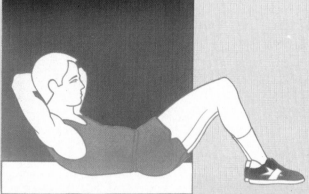

Abdominals/3: From the same starting position, clasp your hands behind your neck, keeping your arms close by your head as you raise your upper back. Holding for at least 30 seconds indicates that your abdominal strength is good.

Abdominals/4: Clasp your hands behind your neck, this time keeping your elbows out to the sides as you lift your upper back. If you can hold this position for at least 30 seconds, the strength of your abdominal muscles is excellent.

Quadriceps: With your back against a wall and your feet about two feet in front of you, slide down so your thighs and calves form a 45- to 90-degree angle. Holding for 30 seconds is fair. Less than 30 seconds is poor; longer is good.

Back extensors: Lie face down with your arms at your sides. Raise your upper torso; hold. If you can sustain this position for one minute, your strength is fair; less than this amount of time is considered poor, and longer is good.

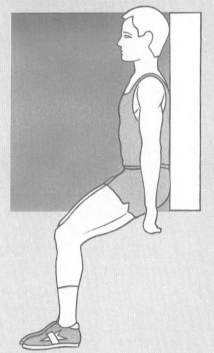

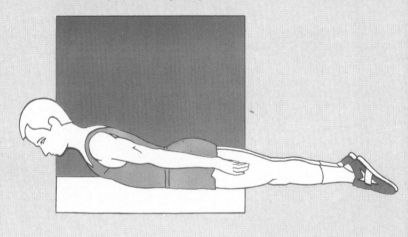

Is Your Posture a Problem?

Posture plays an important role in back care. Aligning your spine correctly allows your abdominal and back muscles to support the back with optimal effectiveness. Conversely, improper alignment strains certain muscles while leaving others underused. Thus, postural improvements must accompany back-strengthening exercises for those exercises to be effective.

Evaluating your posture as shown at right is the first step toward improving it. Stand sideways in front of a mirror in your natural posture, either nude or in form-fitting exercise clothes. Compare your alignment to the standing image. Then sit sideways in front of the mirror and make the same comparison. You will have to turn your head, but doing so will not disrupt your posture from the neck down.

Another way to evaluate the way you stand is to check the soles of your shoes for patterns of wear, as indicated below.

If your posture departs from the ideals shown at right, perform the exercises on pages 72-93, which are designed to encourage changes in longstanding postural habits.

Look at the sole of an exercise or walking shoe you have worn for at least a few weeks. Any wear patterns similar to those shown on the shoe at right indicates faulty posture. Excess wear on the inside of your shoe is due to pronation, an inward rotation of the foot. On the outside of the soles, wear is from supination, an outward rotation. While the proper shoes may alleviate some rotation problems, postural improvements can provide more lasting benefits.

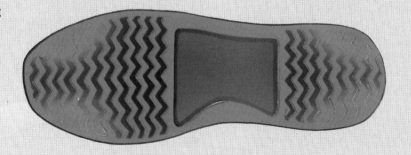

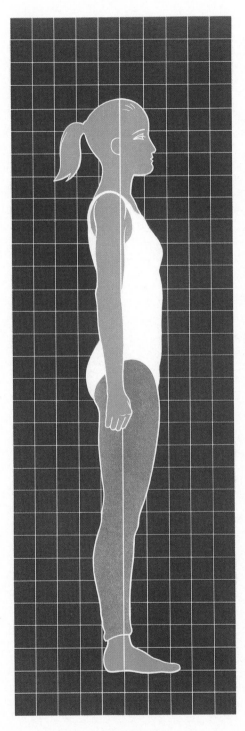

When standing in front of a mirror *(left)*, imagine that a plumb line has been dropped through the center of your head through the front of your earlobe, the front of your shoulder, the center of your hip, behind your kneecap and in front of your ankle-bone. There should be gentle inward curves at your neck and lower back, and a gentle outward curve at your upper back.

When you are sitting *(below)*, the plumb line should pass through the same points and out the center of your hips. There should not be an excessive curve in your lower back.

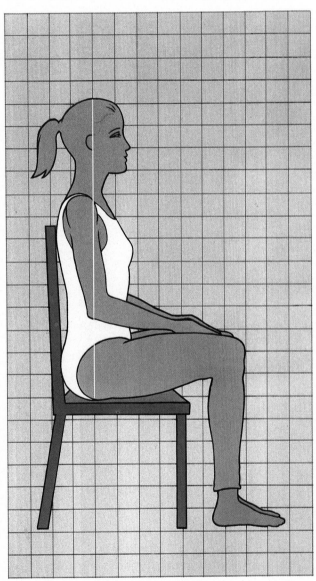

Help for a Bad Back

The majority of back-pain victims are relieved to learn that the trouble is muscular and responds to simple, readily available therapies: bed rest, aspirin and, eventually, an exercise program of stretching and strengthening. For a small minority of sufferers, though, other forms of treatment are essential. The chart below lists some of the choices, from braces and supports, a basic treatment, to surgery, the most risky.

You should consult a physician if you have a backache that does not improve after two days of bed rest, coupled with aspirin or ibuprofen taken every four hours. Your physician will examine you to verify that you have no structural problem or disease. If you need to see a medical specialist, your doctor may refer you to an orthopedist, who specializes in problems of the muscles and bones;

Back Treatment Guide

ACUPUNCTURE

This traditional Chinese treatment, which involves inserting thin needles in the body at certain points, offers relief to some sufferers: In one survey, 54 percent of those undergoing acupuncture reported less pain. Western physicians are not sure how acupuncture works, but one hypothesis is that the needles affect the central nervous system, blocking the transmission of pain impulses.

BRACES AND SUPPORTS

Corsets, braces and back supports can be helpful during the acute stages of back pain, or they may serve as a preventive measure if you are prone to back problems and know you are in for a physically demanding day. These items support your back and maintain your posture. Ultimately, however, muscles should be doing this job, and using artificial support for long periods weakens the muscles, so the treatment becomes self-defeating.

DRUGS

If the pain is severe, your physician may prescribe a strong painkiller like Demerol or codeine, plus an aspirin or other anti-inflammatory drug. The newer types of anti-inflammatory drugs often have proved no more effective than aspirin or a combination of aspirin and codeine, while producing more side effects. Some doctors also prescribe muscle relaxants, such as Valium or Flexeril. Since these compounds and some painkillers have a sedative effect, keep your activity to a minimum while you are taking them. At most, the drugs will lessen the pain during the acute phase of an attack. Some drugs are addictive and physicians are reluctant to prescribe them for long periods.

ELECTRICAL STIMULATION

Also called TENS for Transcutaneous Electrical Nerve Stimulation, this treatment sends mild electrical current to contracted muscle areas, or "trigger points," that send pain radiating to other sites. A tiny battery-powered TENS device can be worn under your clothing, and you can activate it when pain strikes. Although its effects are not understood fully, the temporary relief that TENS provides may be due to the ability of the electrical current to interfere with the body's pain perception mechanisms. (Manual stimulation of trigger points is demonstrated on pages 116-117.)

GRAVITY BOOTS AND INVERSION DEVICES

Hanging upside down in gravity boots or some other kind of inversion system is actually a kind of traction, and some back-pain sufferers find it relaxing. Some proponents suggest that by widening the space between the vertebrae, inversion relieves pressure on the spinal discs. However, because the bottoms-up position elevates blood pressure and may increase pressure in the eyes, it should be avoided by anyone with hypertension or glaucoma.

a physiatrist, who practices rehabilitative medicine; or a neurologist, an expert in nerve disorders.

For a muscular problem that does not respond to rest and aspirin or another analgesic, you might want to consult a chiropractor, a nonmedical specialist who diagnoses pain and muscular disorders as manifestations of spinal misalignments, and treats conditions with manipulation. Other nonmedical specialists who treat back problems include physical therapists, acupuncturists or massage therapists.

If your back pain persists after you have tried a variety of treatments, you may want to explore services offered by a pain clinic. These centers help people cope with persistent, intractable pain by using such approaches and techniques as biofeedback, meditation, visualization, psychotherapy and hypnosis.

INJECTIONS	Physicians sometimes inject anti-inflammatory drugs, most commonly cortisone, or local anesthetics into the sore muscles of back-pain victims who have not responded to more conservative treatments. Cortisone injections can be beneficial for severe pain, and some practitioners believe that anesthetics — mainly Xylocaine or Procaine — can break the pain cycle and relieve spasm when injected into the affected muscle. Some patients have gained relief when their ruptured discs are injected with an enzyme derived from papaya. Called chymopapain, the enzyme may be able to dissolve the protruding part of the disc.
MANUAL THERAPIES	Back-pain victims who responded to a recent survey reported that both massage and chiropractic manipulation produced significant, if temporary, relief. Swedish massage, which involves soothing, gliding motions, helped 66 percent of those who tried it. Shiatsu, Japanese pressure-point therapy which works deeper in the muscles, helped 79 percent, including some who found little relief elsewhere. (A home massage routine is shown on pages 118-123.) Chiropractic manipulation of the spine aided 56 percent. In another study of back-pain sufferers divided into two groups, 50 percent of the group who underwent chiropractic manipulation were pain-free a week after treatment, compared with 27 percent of those treated with bed rest and painkillers. However, physicians warn that you should not receive treatment from a chiropractor if you have a ruptured or herniated disc; sciatica, a nerve problem that affects the legs, hips and buttocks; or any disease of the spine.
SURGERY	Today surgery is generally advised for fewer than 5 percent of sufferers, and then only as a last resort. Even ruptured discs frequently heal without surgery, according to a number of studies. Typically, surgery is undertaken only if a ruptured disc or bone spur impinges far enough on a nerve to cause sciatic leg pain with accompanying numbness and muscular weakness.
TRACTION	When you are placed in traction, a mechanical apparatus that may include harnesses, straps, pulleys and weights in effect pulls the upper and lower parts of your body in opposite directions. Traction stretches the back muscles and ligaments, and some proponents believe that it opens up space for the discs. Although most people are hospitalized to undergo traction, a number of devices are designed for home use. As a rule, this therapy provides short-term relief, and once you stop using traction, your vertebrae will gradually return to their former positions.

Dealing with Back Attacks

Episodes of back spasm are usually immobilizing as well as painful; once they strike, there is not much you can do but lie down. Fortunately, while some attacks come on suddenly, most attacks are preceded by telltale twinges and excessive back fatigue. In fact, except for traumatic injury, nearly all back spasms mark the culmination of problems that have been growing worse for some time. Learning to respond to your back's signals can help prevent full-fledged spasms before they develop.

The following sequence is designed to prevent or reduce pain by relaxing your back-supporting muscles and lengthening your spine, thus relieving compression of the vertebrae. When you do have back pain, first lie down to eliminate pressure on the spine. After a period of rest, gentle stretching will help relax back muscles and take pressure off the nerves.

These exercises should be done slowly and gently. They are designed to help your back feel better; do not perform any movement that causes pain. If your back pain is so severe that you cannot perform any of these exercises, consult your physician.

The two exercises on page 29 can be performed when back pain strikes but you have no place to lie down to recuperate. By reducing the curve in your lower back, they relieve pressure from too much standing or walking.

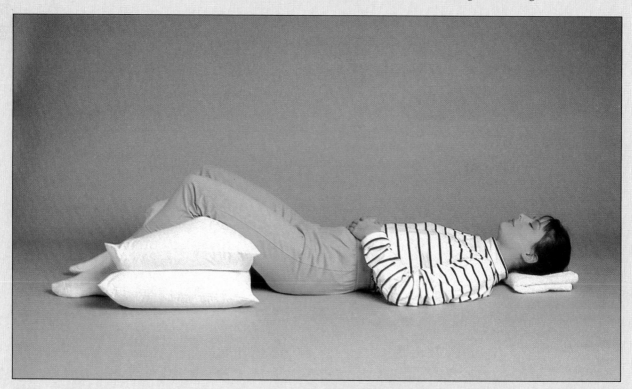

Whenever your back bothers you, this position is ideal for resting and relieving pressure on your spine. Place a small pillow or rolled-up towel under your head to prevent it from tipping back. Raise your knees by putting one or two large pillows underneath to keep your back flat. Close your eyes and relax for at least 20 minutes before continuing the sequence.

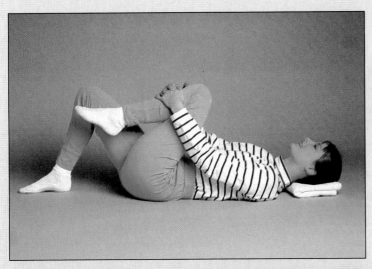

Leave the small pillow or towel under your head. Remove the large pillow but keep your knees bent. Grasp your left knee with both hands and pull it gently to your chest. Lower and repeat with your other leg.

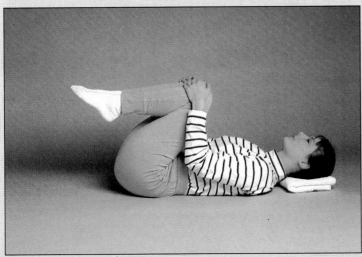

Remain lying down with both knees bent and your feet flat on the floor. Keeping your back flat, grasp your knees and gently pull them toward your chest. Lower your knees.

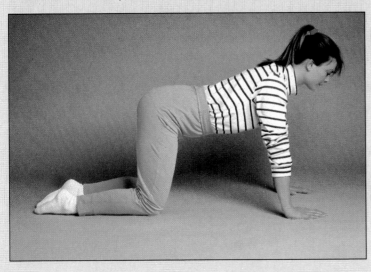

Carefully roll over onto your stomach and raise yourself onto your hands and knees, with your arms shoulder-width apart and your knees hip-width apart. Then gently arch your back.

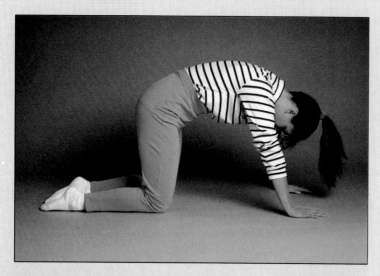

Stay on your hands and knees and drop your head between your arms. Round your back, allowing it to curve upward.

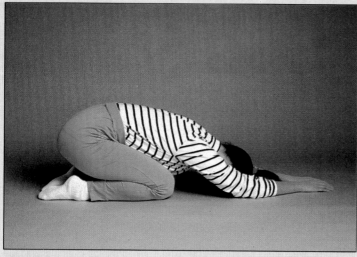

With your legs about two inches apart, lower your buttocks to your heels, folding your chest onto your thighs and dropping your forehead to the floor. Keep your arms extended in front of your head.

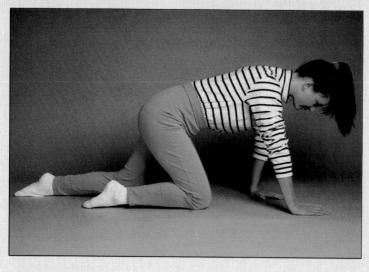

Keep your head down and your neck and back straight and raise yourself onto your hands and knees. Using alternate arms and legs, crawl a few feet forward, then retrace your movement backward.

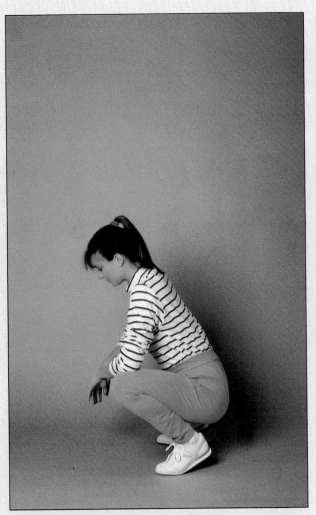

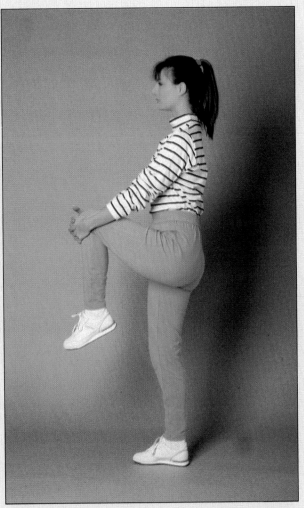

From an upright position, lower yourself into a squat. Although it is not necessary, you may rest your heels on the floor if it is comfortable. Keep your back and neck aligned and rest your elbows on your knees. Hold for approximately 30 seconds.

From a standing position, bend your left leg and raise it to hip height or higher. Clasp your hands around your knee and pull the leg toward your chest slightly. Hold for several seconds; lower and repeat with your other leg.

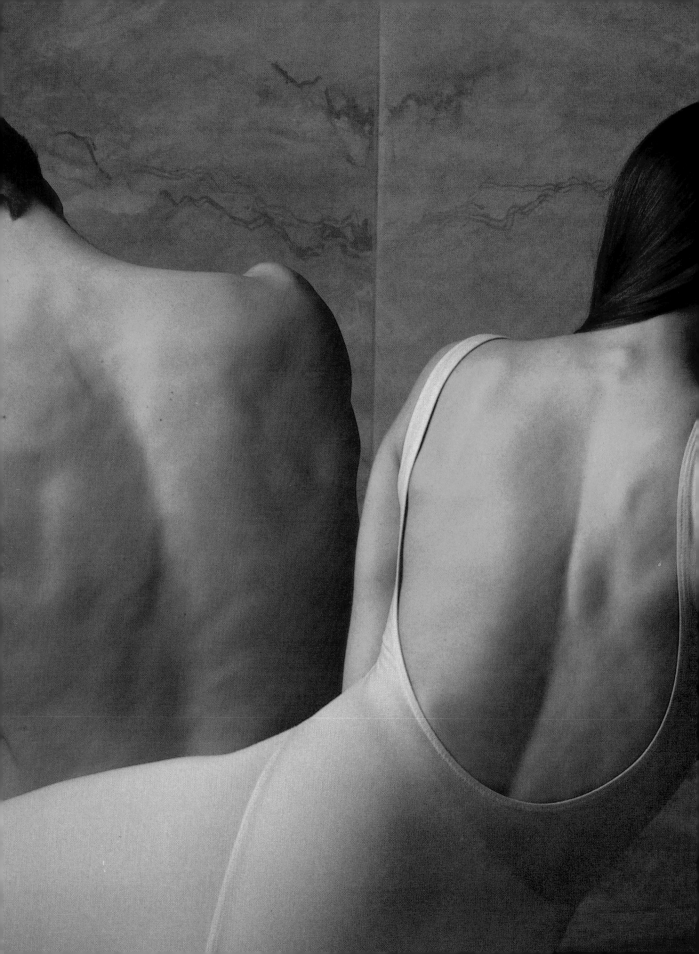

CHAPTER TWO

Building a Better Back

*A progressive strengthening
and stretching routine
for insurance against backache*

The principle that strong, flexible muscles are the best defense against most types of injury proves especially valid where the back is concerned. An exercise program aimed at strengthening the muscles that support the back is one effective step you can take for preventing lower back problems.

Research has confirmed that the large majority of back-pain sufferers can blame their discomfort on muscular weaknesses. In one study, only 17 percent of a group of back-pain patients showed signs of structural problems or pathology. But when the entire group of 3,000 people was given six standard tests to measure the strength and flexibility of the muscles that support the back, 83 percent of them failed one or more test. In a separate study of 174 patients who had made significant improvements in the same tests, 88 percent reported a decrease in back pain accompanying the muscular changes.

Several recent studies have shown that the proper type of exercises, when performed regularly, can contribute to restoring strength and flexibility in a back that has been injured or weakened by strain, sprain or spasm. One such study involved 12,000 men and women enrolled in a YMCA program to combat lower back pain. Working out both at home and at their local Y, participants engaged daily in strengthening, relaxation and flexibility exercises for six weeks. Four out of five participants — including those who had suffered back pain for up to 15 years — reported that their pain had vanished or was alleviated by the end of the program. Whether a participant had previously tried another form of treatment had no significant impact on any improvement that occurred. Of the nearly 600 participants who had undergone back surgery but enrolled because of continuing pain, those who exercised daily for more than a half-hour showed more dramatic improvement than those who worked out less often.

Exercises targeted at strengthening the back focus on three groups of muscles. The abdominals, latissimus dorsi and obliques support the torso itself. The erector spinae muscles, called the back extensors, extend the length of the spine and connect to the vertebrae, providing direct support and stability for the spine. The quadriceps, large four-part muscles along the fronts of the thighs, stabilize the pelvis.

Of these muscle groups, the abdominals are the most important for back support, functioning much like powerful rubber bands to connect your upper and lower body and transfer force between them. When well conditioned, these muscles, which run diagonally, horizontally and vertically, create the equivalent of a muscular girdle that protects the internal organs and keeps the lower back from overarching into the swayback position. Aerobic workouts, weight training and other forms of exercise often fail to condition the abdominals. One study of Canadian athletes who competed in the 1976 Olympics found that they had relatively weak abdominal muscles. Some were unable to perform more than one bent-knee sit-up.

Weak abdominal muscles put the back in double jeopardy. Not only do lax abdominals fail to provide adequate support but, because they are less able to resist the pull of the body's weight on the spine, they may actually create back strain. Although they are not designed for the task of keeping your spine upright, the spinal muscles are forced to assume most of the burden. Performing abdominal-strengthening exercises will help alleviate this overload on the spine.

Strong back extensors can absorb much of the stress of everyday movements like leaning forward. However, these important muscles tend to be misused in people who suffer chronic back trouble. The lack of torso support provided by weak abdominals is often compensated for by the extensors. Similarly, the back extensors are commonly used for lifting — a function more appropriately relegated to the quadriceps. Such inappropriate demands stress the extensors, making them prone to sprain, which can result in painful backaches.

The quadriceps, among the largest and most powerful muscles in the body, supply much of the momentum for running, jumping and all other forms of forward movement. When appropriately used, they

Muscles that Maintain Your Back

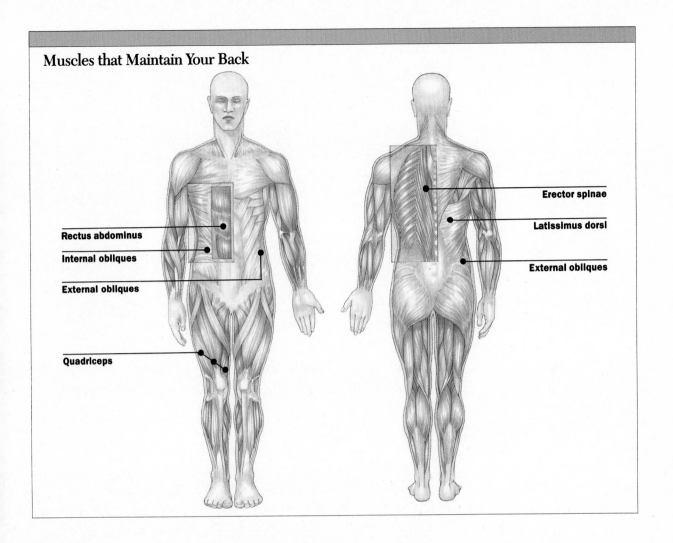

Rectus abdominus

Internal obliques

External obliques

Quadriceps

Erector spinae

Latissimus dorsi

External obliques

have the capacity to relieve the back of much of the burden of lifting heavy objects. Lifting and bending should utilize the quadriceps, rather than the muscles of the back. Strengthening your quadriceps will allow you to use them more comfortably for lifting.

Physicians advise that you should not begin an exercise program if you are suffering intense or disabling back pain. Wait until the injured tissues have had a chance to heal; exercise may aggravate the problem rather than relieve it. The following workout incorporates both strengthening and flexibility exercises. The strengthening sequence is divided into basic, moderate and advanced exercises. If you have not exercised regularly in some time, start with the minimal number of repetitions. Do not advance to the next level until you can comfortably perform the maximum number. Be aware of how your back adapts itself to the exercises and stop if you feel any pain. Always work slowly and smoothly, avoiding sudden jerking movements. For the best results, perform the range-of-motion and stretching exercises daily, and the strengthening exercises at least three times a week.

Range of Motion Routine/1

Building back strength demands a comprehensive fitness program aimed at increasing both muscle strength and muscle flexibility, as well as maximizing range of motion within the joints. The exercises in this chapter target all three of these areas.

The exercises are intended to be done as a routine. The warm-up consists of the range-of-motion sequences on these two pages and the following four. These exercises enhance flexibility in the hip joints, which connect the pelvis to the legs, as well as in the vertebrae themselves. Strengthening and stretching sequences make up the remainder of the chapter.

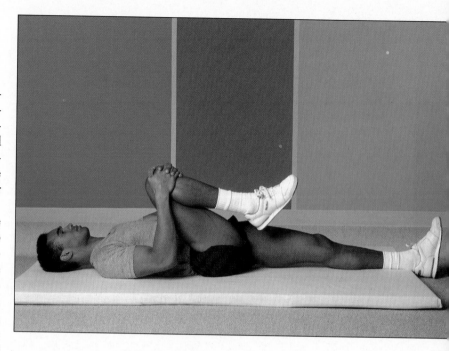

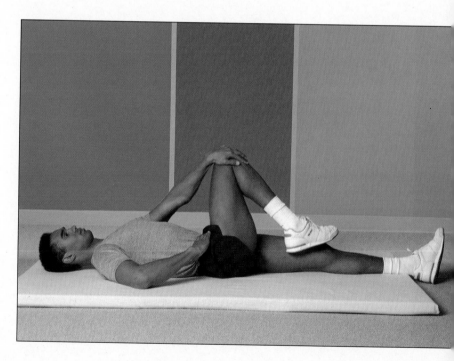

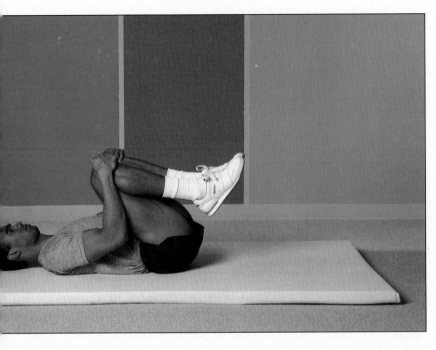

To increase hip joint range of motion, lie on your back with your legs extended. Bend your right knee and grasp it with your hands, bringing it toward your chest *(far left)*. Hold 10 seconds, then lower. Repeat three to five times with the right knee. Switch knees and repeat. Then bring up both knees and grasp them for 10 seconds *(near left)*; lower. Repeat three to five times.

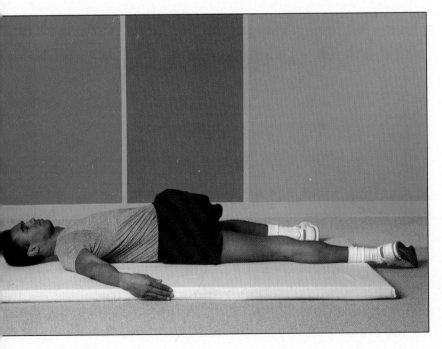

Lying down with your legs extended, bend your right knee so that your right foot touches your left knee. Place your right hand at your right hip to make sure it is flat and grasp your right knee with your other hand *(far left)*. Next, keeping your shoulders flat, rotate your right hip as you pull your knee across your body with your left hand *(left)*. Hold 10 seconds, return and repeat three to five times. Switch legs and repeat.

Range of Motion
Routine/2

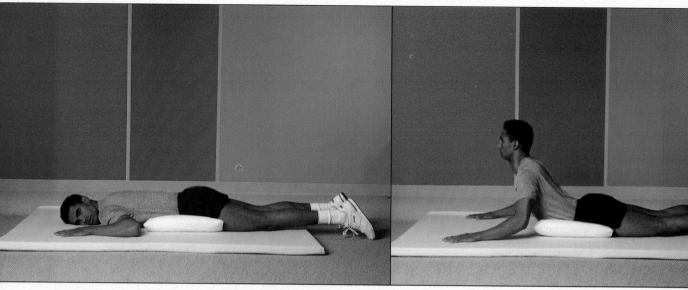

To improve the range of motion in your lower back, lie on your abdomen with a pillow beneath you and your elbows bent so that your hands are about six inches in front of your shoulders *(above)*. Pushing up with your arms, raise your upper body so that it curves gently to form a "C" *(right)*. Keep your elbows slightly bent. Lower. Perform 10 repetitions.

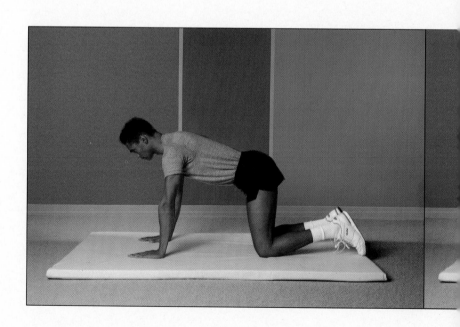

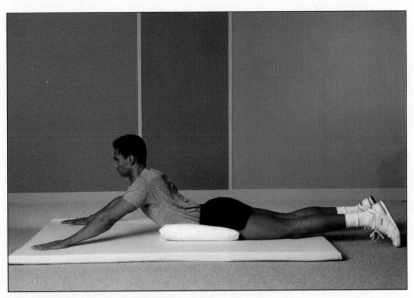

If the exercise opposite causes pain, try this variation. Place your hands 12 inches in front of your shoulders and push up, straightening your arms.

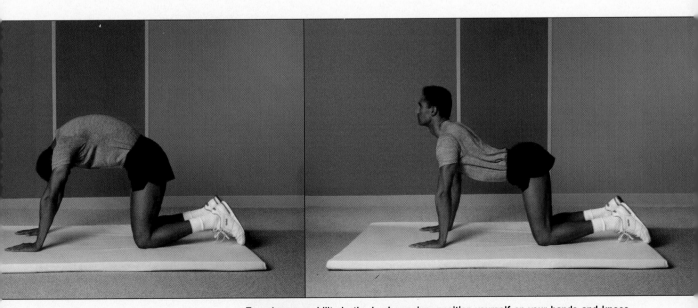

To enhance mobility in the lumbar spine, position yourself on your hands and knees with your back flat *(far left)*. Shift your weight slightly backward, tucking your head and rounding your back upward *(center)*. Then shift your weight forward, arching your back and lifting your head *(above)*. Hold each position for 10 seconds and repeat the sequence five times.

Range of Motion Routine/3

For greater mobility in the thoracic spine, rest on your knees and forearms, with your entire spine straight, including the neck *(right)*. Shift your weight forward, arching your back slightly *(center)*. Then shift your weight backward, rounding your back and dropping your head *(bottom)*. Hold each position for 10 seconds; repeat five times.

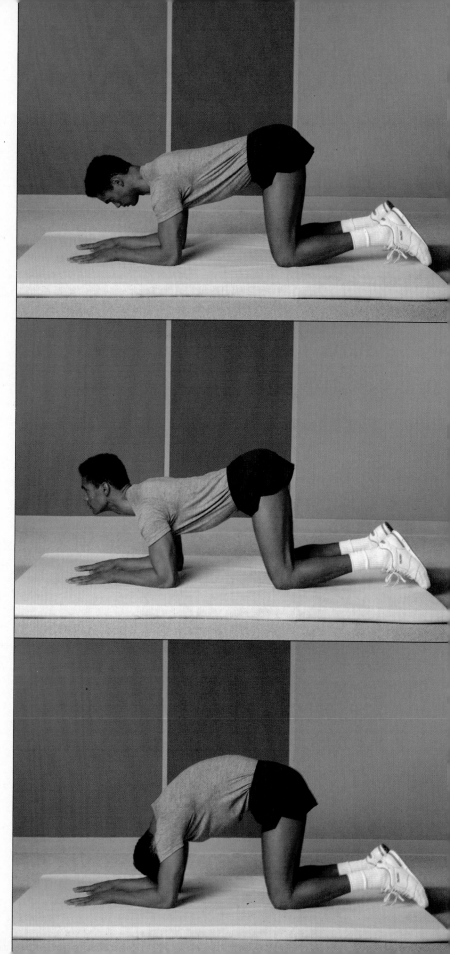

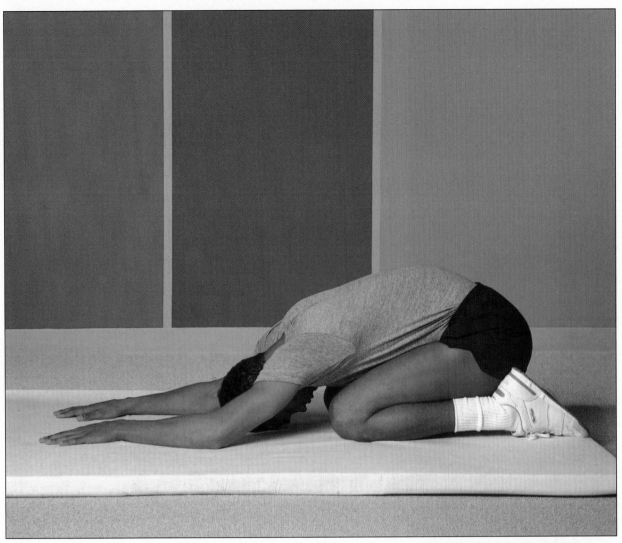

Kneel with your legs together. Shift your weight backward trying to rest your buttocks on your heels. Then tuck your head and drop your chest to your thighs *(above)*. Keep your arms extended in front of you. Hold for up to 30 seconds.

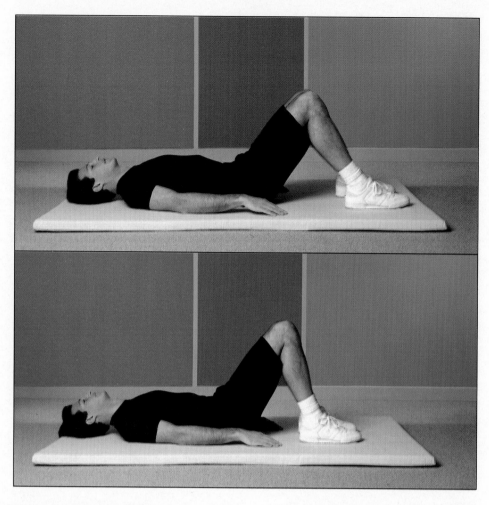

Strengtheners and Stretches

Maximizing the strength and flexibility of the back-supporting musculature is the cornerstone of back fitness. The major muscles supporting the back are the back extensors and lattisimus dorsi in the back, the abdominal muscles and the quadriceps muscles at the front of the thigh. (*See box, page 33.*)

The exercises in the remainder of this chapter focus on these muscle groups. The strengthening exercises are divided into three groups: basic, intermediate and advanced. Unless you were in the highest performance categories on the strong-back test on pages 20-21, you should probably start with the basic routine. Even if

you are generally fit, your back-supporting musculature will be weak unless you have targeted it in a training program.

If you experience pain while performing these exercises, reduce the repetitions or drop back a level. When more than one set is indicated, pause for 15-30 seconds between sets. Particularly at the advanced level, these exercises are quite rigorous. The routines will not only strengthen your back but will tone your midsection, making you look slimmer.

Finish your back workout with the stretching routine on pages 56-61 and the three neck stretches on pages 62-65.

BASIC STRENGTHENERS: To tighten your upper abdominals, lie on your back with your knees bent and your arms at your sides *(top)*. Rotate your pelvis back, flattening your lower back against the floor to tilt your abdomen upward *(above)*. Focus on the muscles involved, being careful not to tighten your buttocks or lift your ribs. Do two sets of 10, holding for five seconds each.

For lower abdominal strength, lie flat on your back with your arms at your sides *(opposite above)*. Raise your head and lift your arms, rounding your upper back *(opposite)*. You should feel your lower abdominals contract. Hold five seconds; repeat 10 times.

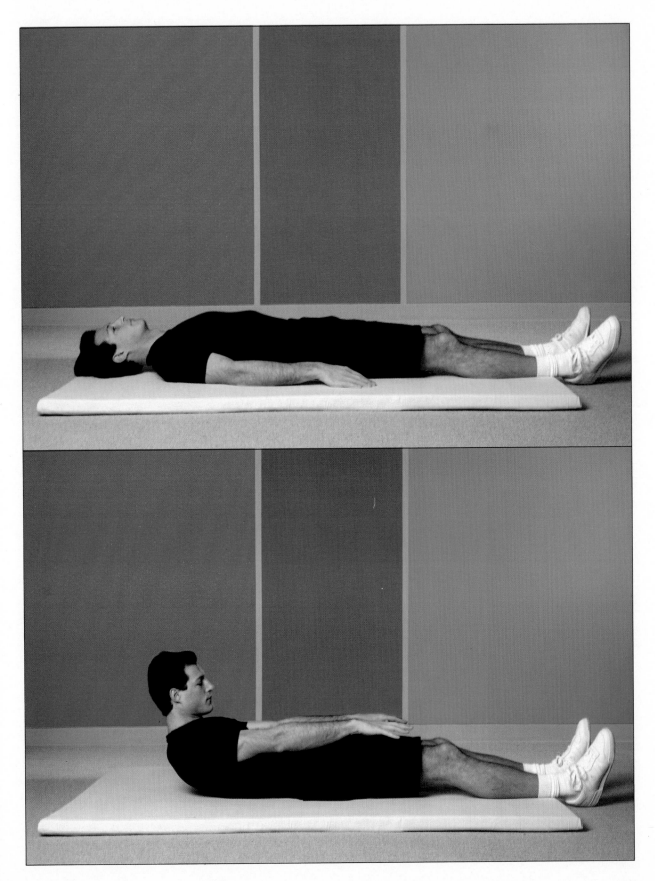

Basic Strengtheners/2

To strengthen the oblique abdominals, which run diagonally, bend your knees while lying on your back. Lift your legs and cross your feet. Cross your hands behind your head *(right)*. Twist your left elbow toward your right knee, raising your upper back *(center);* lower yourself back down. Twist up again to raise your right elbow toward your left knee *(bottom)*. Work up to three sets of 10.

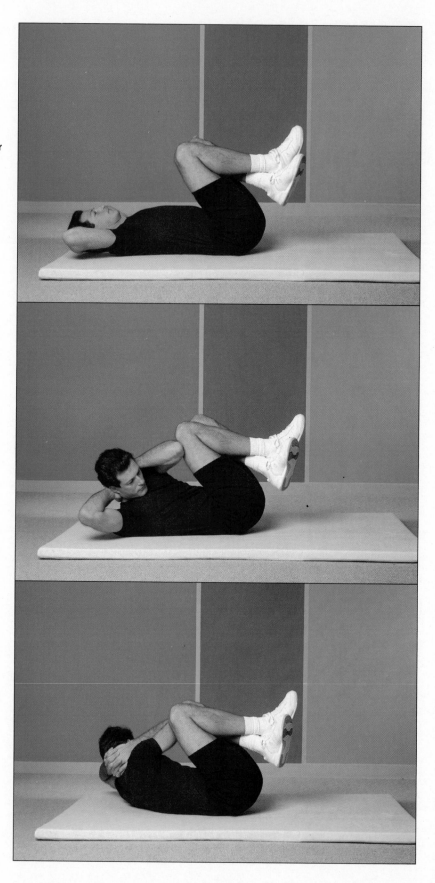

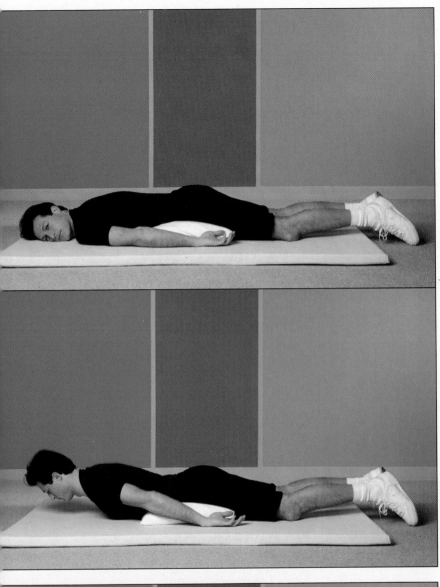

To strengthen your back muscles,
lie prone with a pillow beneath your
abdomen and your arms at your sides
(above). Squeeze your shoulders together
to bring your upper body up slightly *(left)*.
Keep your neck in line with your spine;
lower yourself back down. Perform 10
full repetitions.

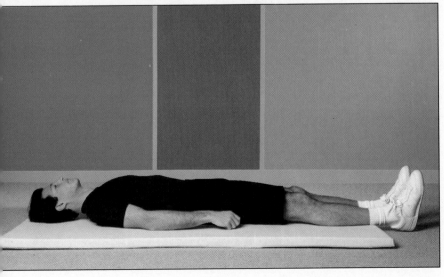

To build up the thigh muscles needed for
proper lifting, lie on your back with your
arms at your sides. Tighten the quadriceps,
or thigh muscles, of your left leg as much
as possible *(left)*. Perform 10 repetitions,
holding for 10 seconds each. Switch legs
and repeat.

43

Basic Strengtheners/3

This exercise uses the test for quadriceps strength on page 20 to build up these muscles. Stand with your back, shoulders and buttocks flat against a wall *(right)*. Move your heels about 12 inches from the wall. Slide down the wall, keeping your back flat, until your knees and thighs are at about a 45-degree angle *(center)*. Stop at this point if your knees hurt; otherwise continue until your legs form a 90-degree angle *(far right)*. Hold your position for 15 seconds; rise and repeat twice. To increase the difficulty, build up to sets of 60 seconds in 10-second increments.

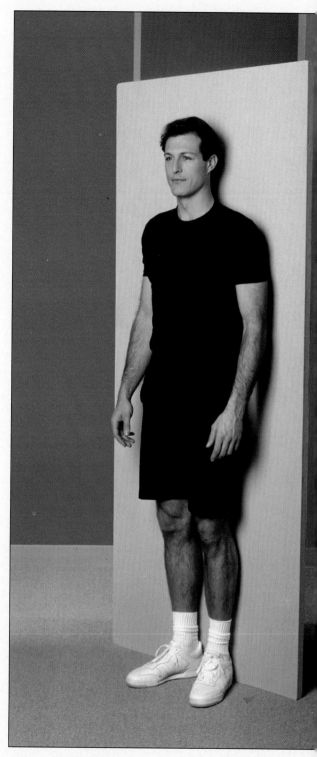

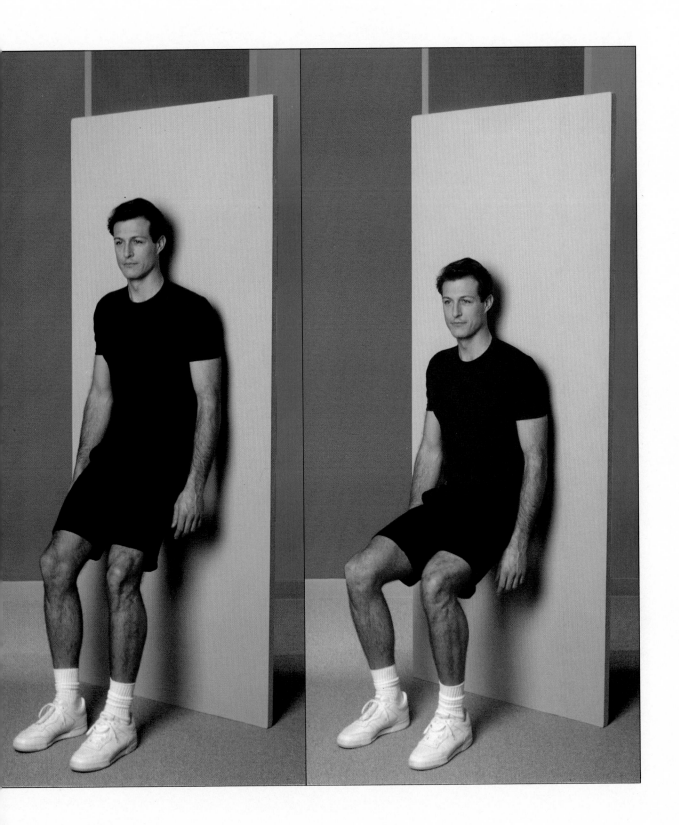

Intermediate Strengtheners/1

To further increase abdominal strength, lie on your back with your knees bent and your feet flat on the floor *(near right)*. Bend your elbows, place your hands at your temples and, keeping your elbows close together, lift your upper back so your shoulder blades come off the mat *(far right)*. Do three sets of 10; work up to sets of 20 repetitions.

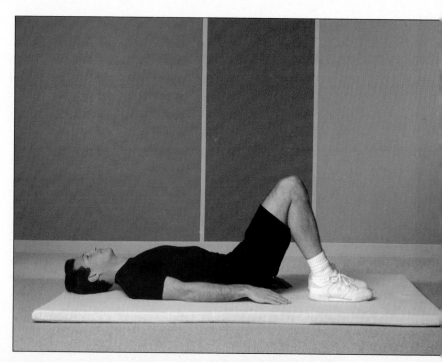

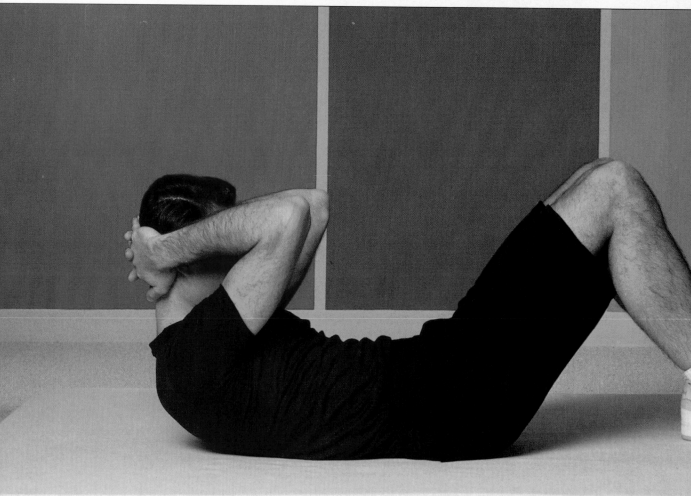

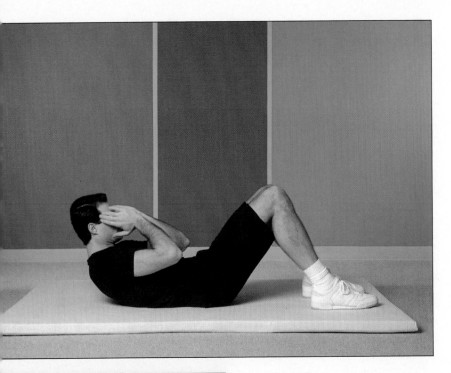

If you have any neck pain, do this variation on the above exercise: Clasp your hands behind your neck for support, keeping your elbows close by your head. Raise your shoulders off the mat.

Intermediate Strengtheners/2

Improve lower abdominal strength by lying on your back with your left knee bent and left foot on the floor, your right knee raised toward your chest *(right)*. Straighten your right knee, pointing the sole of your foot toward the ceiling *(center)*. Slowly lower your right leg, stopping just before your back begins to arch *(bottom)*. Keep your hips down. Hold for 10 seconds; return to the starting position. Be sure to keep your back flat. Perform 10 repetitions for each leg.

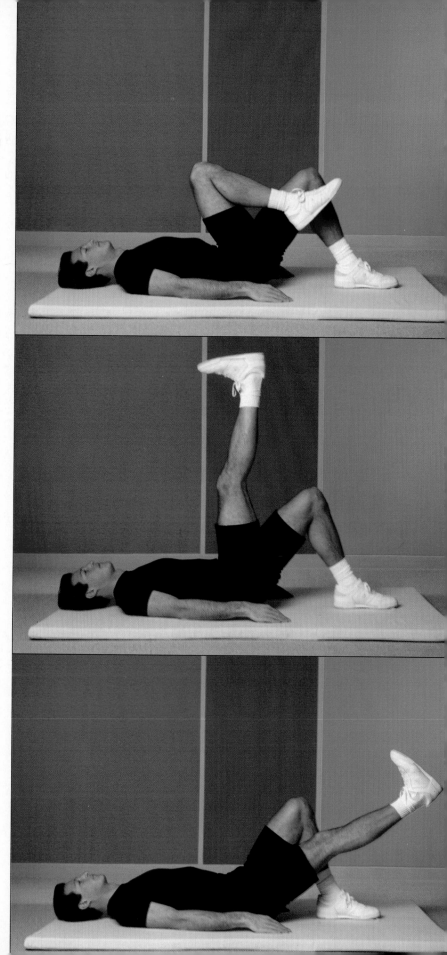

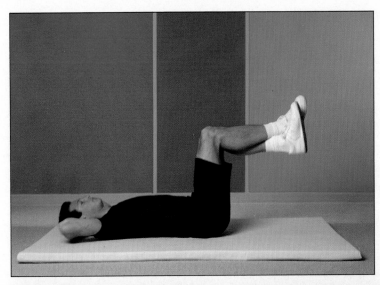

To strengthen the oblique abdominals, lie flat on your back with your legs raised and knees bent to form a 90-degree angle. Cross your ankles and cross your hands under your head *(left)*. Lift your upper back and twist to your right, reaching your left elbow to your right knee *(below)*. Lower and twist to your left. Do three sets of 10.

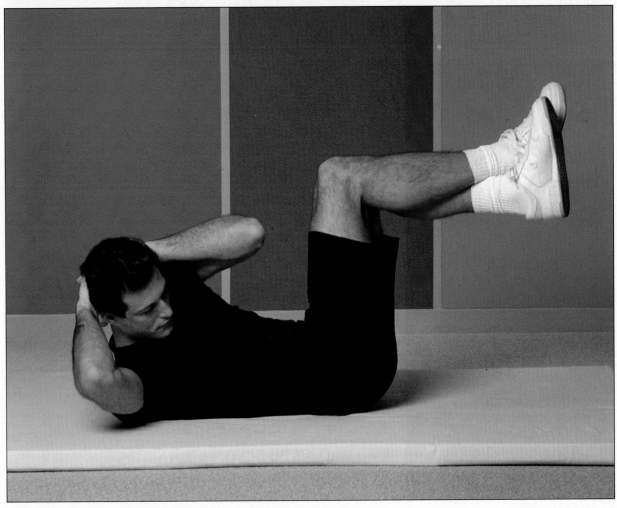

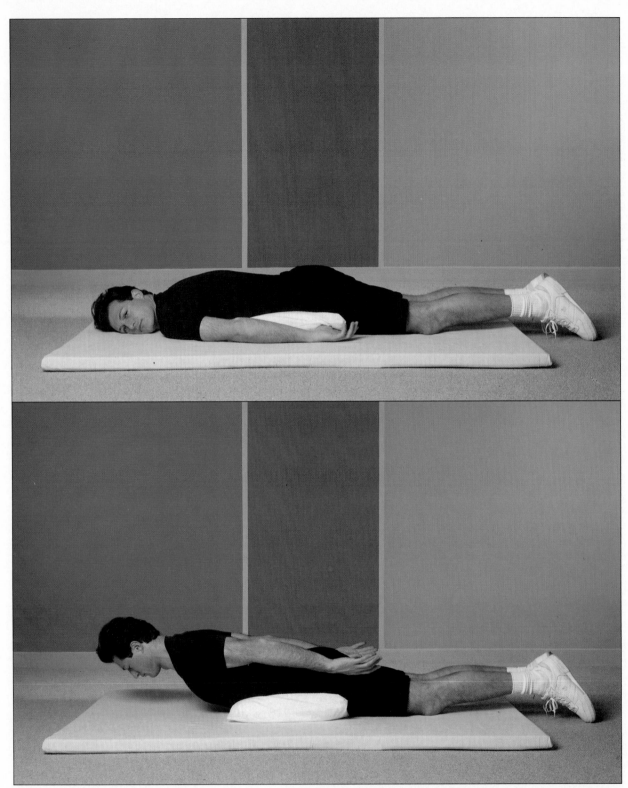

Intermediate Strengtheners/3

Increase the strength of your back muscles by lying prone with your arms at your sides and a pillow beneath you *(top)*. Lift your upper back, raising your arms and your entire upper torso *(above)*. Keep your head in line with your spine. Do two sets of 10 repetitions.

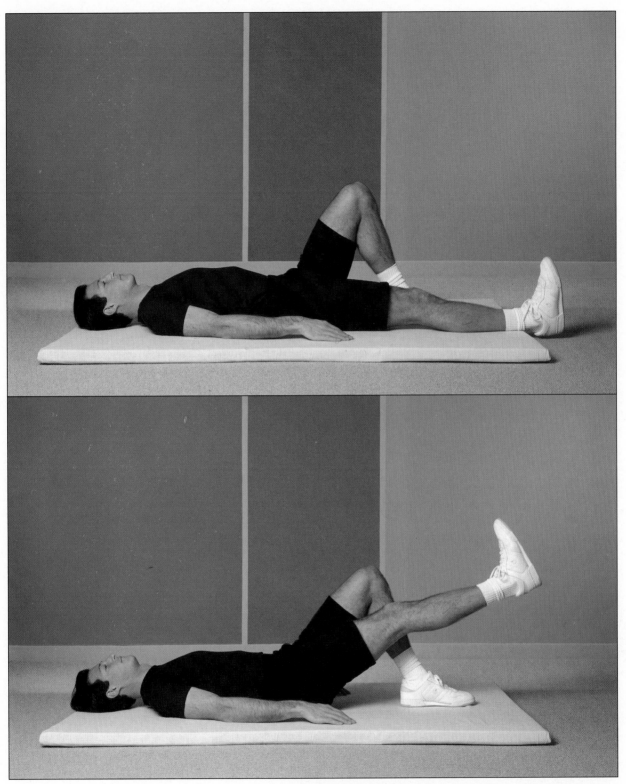

To increase quadriceps strength, lie on your back with your left knee bent and your left foot flat on the floor *(top)*. Raise your right leg about 12 inches or just until your back starts to arch *(above)*. Hold for 10 seconds; lower. Do 15 times, then switch legs.

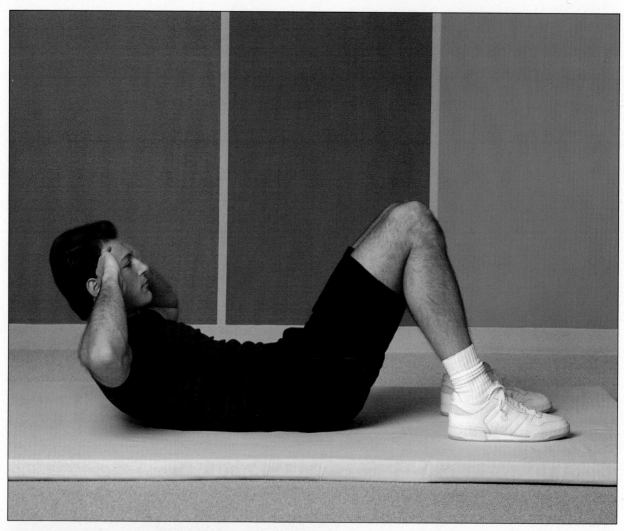

Advanced
Strengtheners/1

To strengthen and tone your upper
abdominals, lie on your back with your
knees and elbows bent and your hands at
your temples *(left)*. Raise your upper
torso, keeping your arms open *(above)*.
Do three sets of 10; work up to 20.

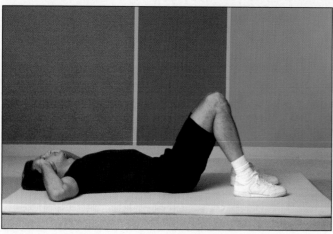

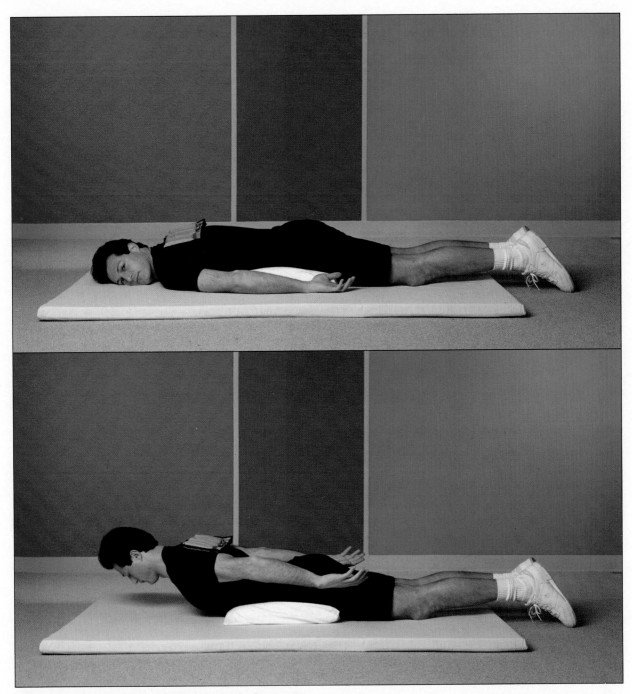

Place a 10-pound cuff weight across your upper back near your
shoulders and lie on your abdomen with a pillow beneath you
(top). Raise your arms and upper torso *(above)*. Do three sets of
10 repetitions.

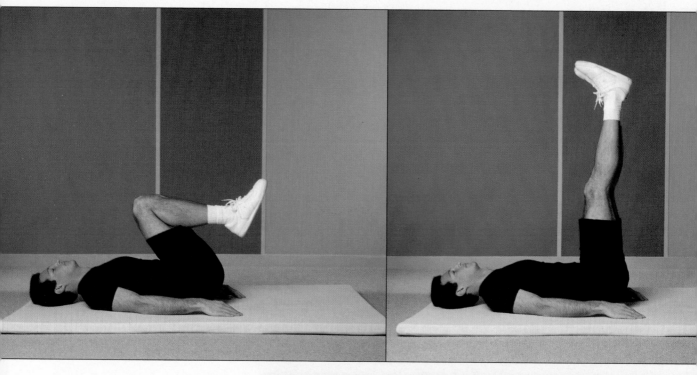

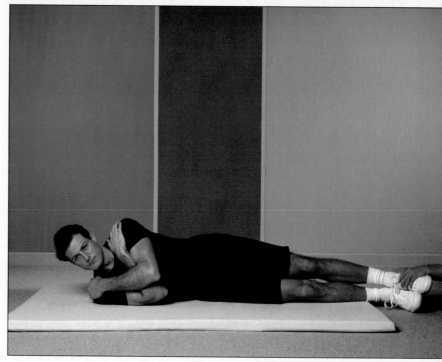

Advanced
Strengtheners/2

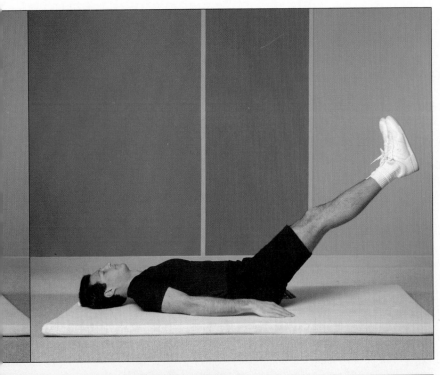

Lie on your back with your arms at your sides. Bend your knees and lift your legs *(far left)*. Straighten your legs *(center)*, then lower them together *(left)*. Stop lowering just before your lower back starts to arch. Use extreme caution to avoid arching your back. Return to the starting position. Beginning with one set of 10 repetitions, work up to two sets of 10 each.

To strengthen both your abdominals and back muscles, lie on your right side and cross your arms in front of you so that your hands grasp your shoulders. Have someone hold your feet or hook them under a heavy piece of furniture *(far left)*. Raise your upper torso *(left)*. Hold momentarily; then lower. Start with five repetitions and work up to 10. Repeat on your left side.

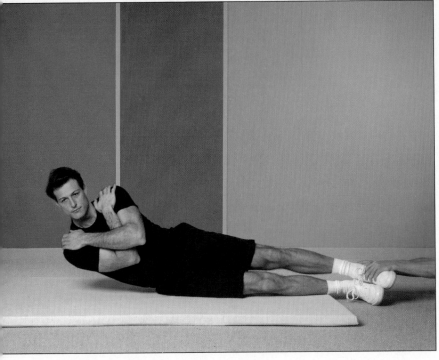

Stretches/1

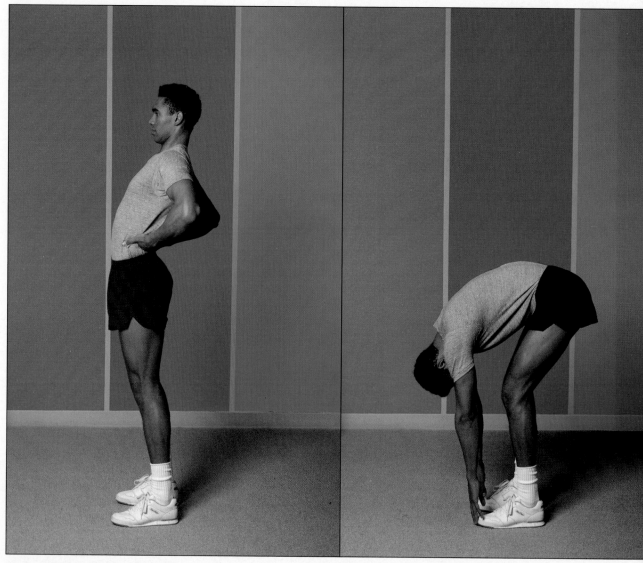

From a standing position, place your hands behind your waist and draw your shoulders together, arching your back *(above)*. Hold briefly, then drop your arms to the floor and slowly bend forward, keeping your back rounded and bending your knees slightly *(right)*. Perform four full repetitions.

To stretch your chest muscles, stand with your feet shoulder-width apart. Grasp a rolled towel or stick behind your back. Slowly raise your arms as far as you can *(right)*. Hold, then lower. Perform four repetitions.

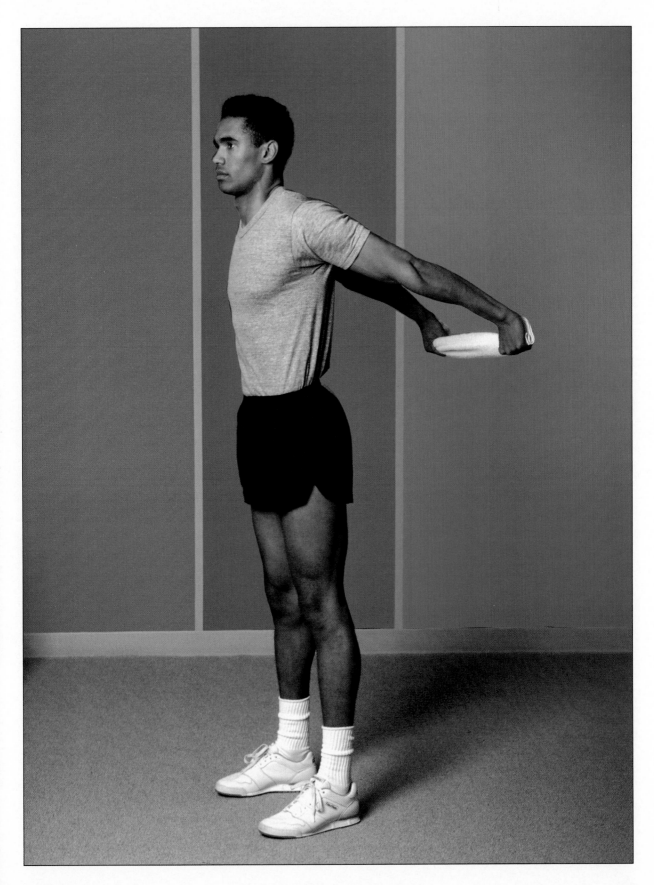

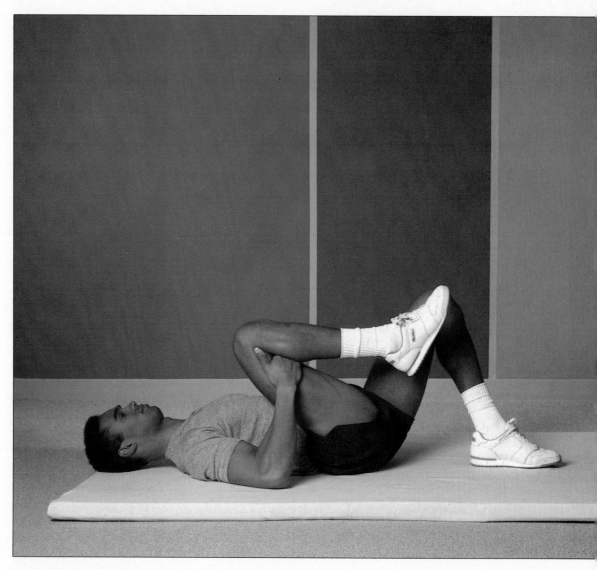

Stretches/2

Lie on your back with both knees bent.
Grasp your right thigh and pull your knee
to your chest *(above)*. Slowly straighten
your leg, keeping your foot relaxed *(above
opposite)*. Return to the second position;
perform four repetitions. Return to the
starting position and switch legs.

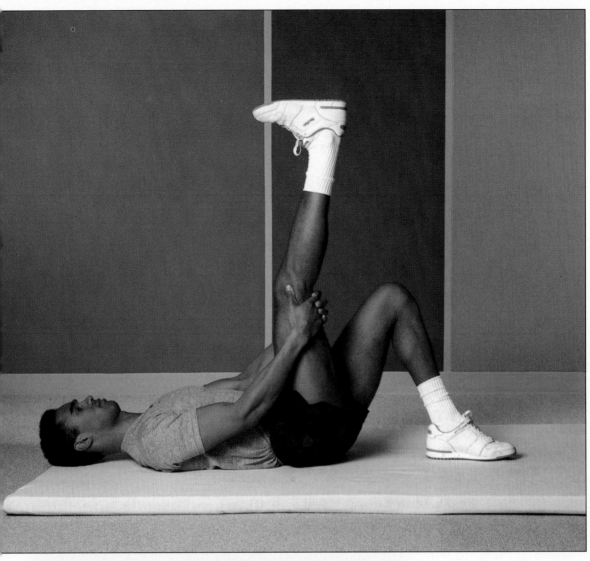

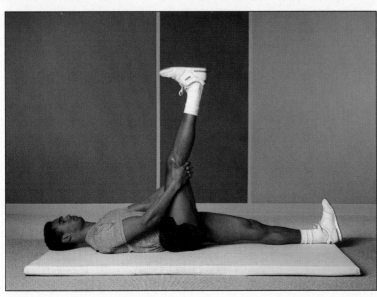

For a more difficult variation on the above exercise, keep your left leg straight when you lift the right, and vice versa.

Stretches/3

Stand at arm's length from a stool or table and extend your left leg behind you. Bend your right knee and, keeping your left leg straight, lean forward, stretching your calf *(right)*. Hold for 10 seconds and relax. Perform four repetitions, then switch legs and repeat.

Lie on your abdomen with a pillow beneath you. Bend your left knee, bringing your foot backward. Grasp it with your left hand and hold momentarily *(below)*. Perform four repetitions, then switch legs and repeat.

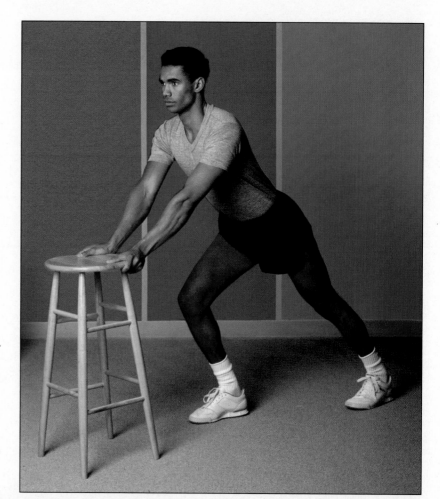

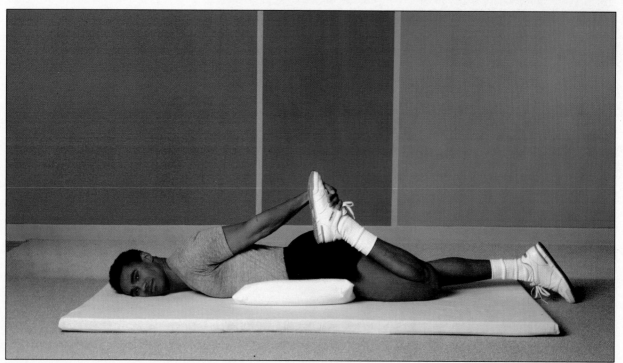

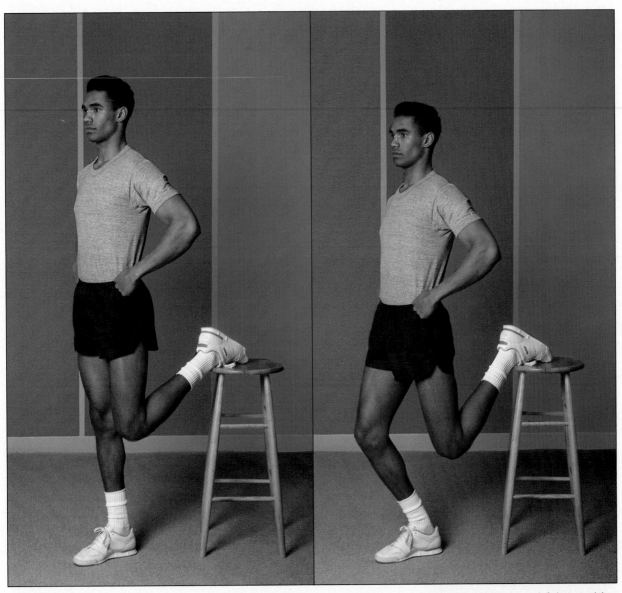

Stand up and bend your left knee, raising your foot and resting it behind you on a high stool or table *(above left)*. Bend your right knee and lower your body *(above)*. Hold, keeping your back straight, then return to the starting position. Perform four repetitions, then switch legs.

Neck Stretches/1

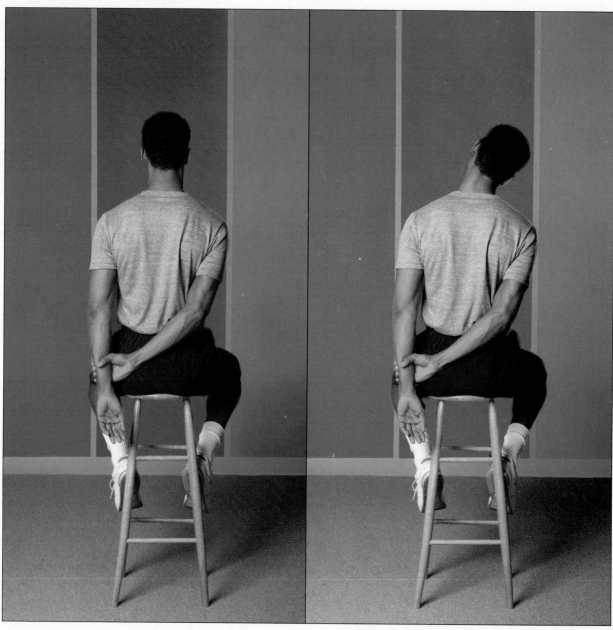

Sit on a stool or a chair with a low back. Keeping your left arm at your side, reach behind you and grasp your left wrist with your right hand *(above left)*. Simultaneously pull down on your left arm and lean your head to the right *(above)*. Return to the first position. Perform four repetitions, then switch arms and repeat.

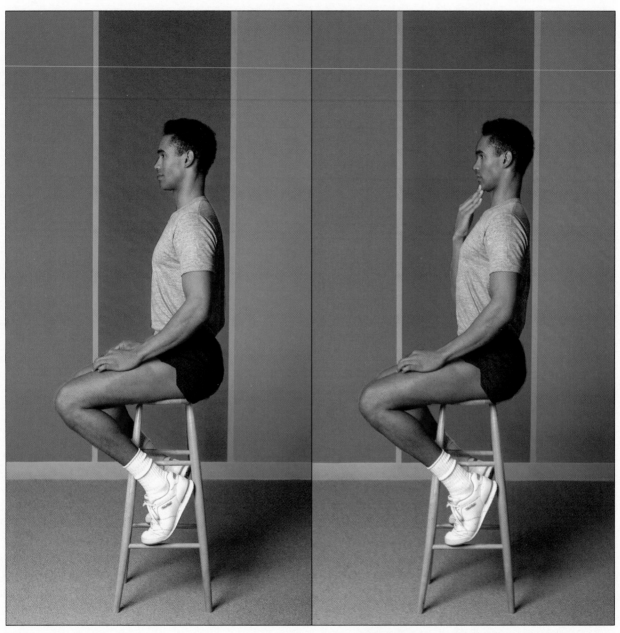

Look ahead as you sit straight on a stool or chair *(above left)*. Slide your head backward, keeping your gaze fixed. Raise your hand to your chin and press your chin inward to increase the stretch to your neck muscles *(above)*. Hold this position momentarily; release. Perform four repetitions.

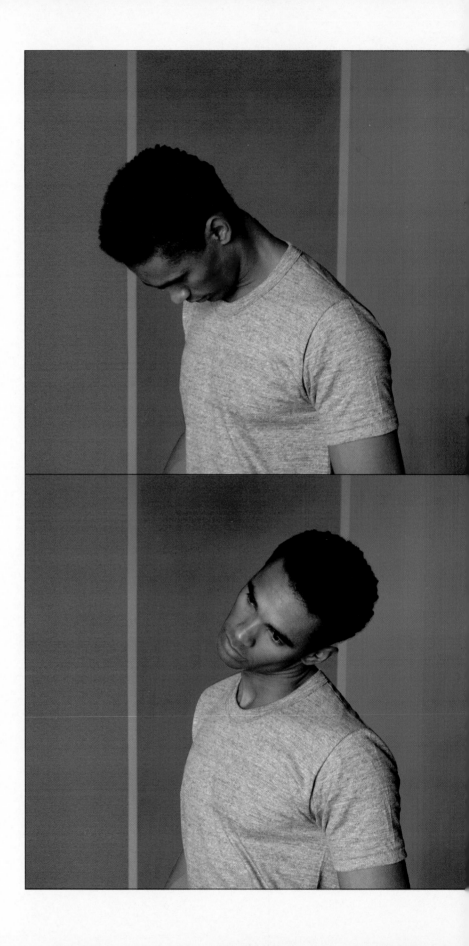

Neck Stretches/2

This exercise can be done from either a sitting or standing position. Clockwise from far left: drop your head to your chest, then slowly rotate it to your right, backward and to your left. Return to the starting position. Perform four repetitions.

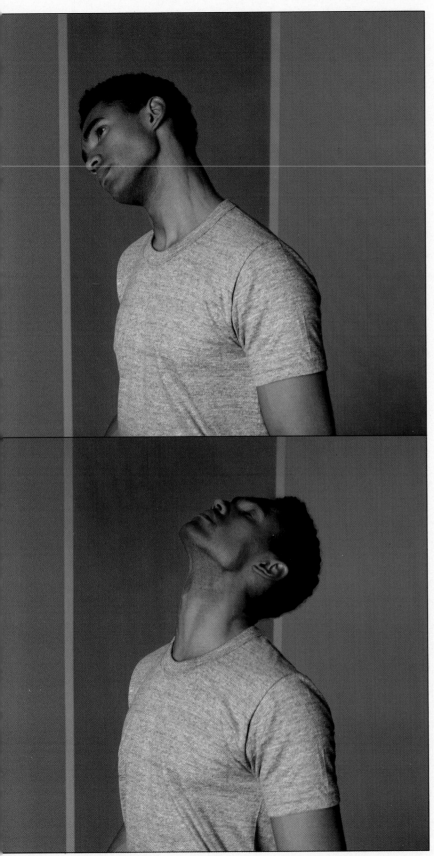

Seated Stretches

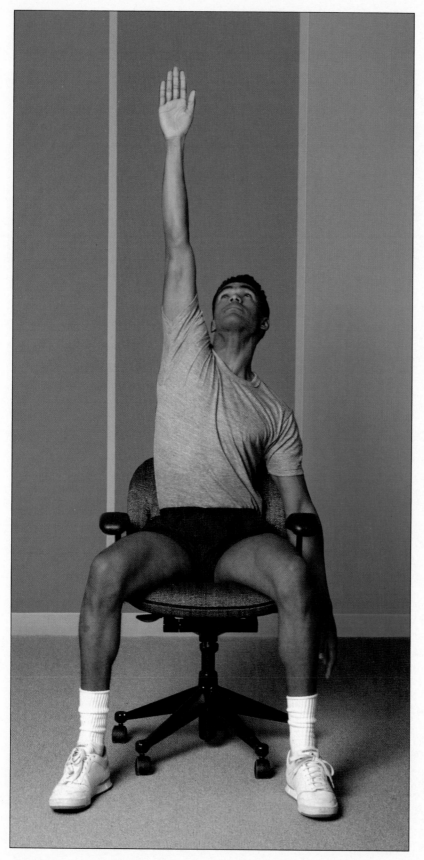

A good deal of the back strain that plagues many office workers develops from long hours of sitting. With prolonged sitting, the back extensor muscles that allow the back to bend become either lengthened or shortened. If you have a desk job, it is imperative to maintain back mobility by standing and walking at frequent intervals during the day.

Additionally, you can perform some stretches right at your desk to maintain joint mobility and to retain muscle flexibility. The exercises on these two pages mimic some of the standing stretches on the previous pages, but they are modified for sitting. They stretch not only the neck muscles but the muscles of both the upper and lower back. Because these exercises take a minimum of time and effort, they can be performed several times throughout the day.

Sit with your back against the back of your chair. Reach straight up from your shoulder with your right arm, looking upward to extend the stretch through your side. Hold, then lower and switch arms. Perform four repetitions.

To increase back mobility, sit with your back firmly against the back of your chair. Clockwise from top left: place your hands on the back of your chair and stretch backward, then drop your hands to the floor and lean forward with your head between your knees. Come back up and place your hands behind your waist, arching your back forward, then grasp the arm or side of the chair and turn to your left; switch sides and turn to your right. Perform four repetitions.

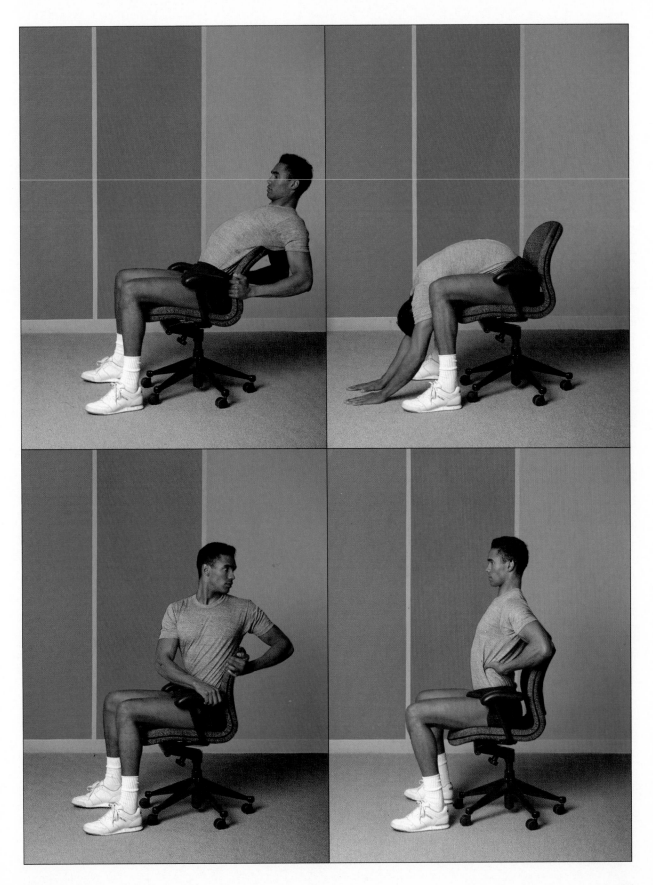

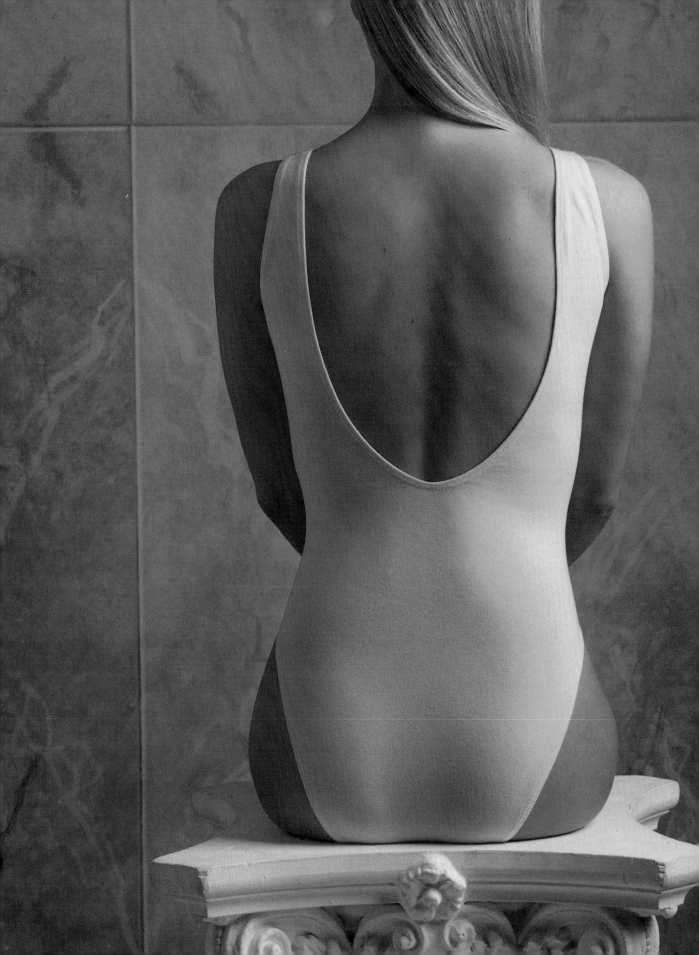

CHAPTER THREE

Posture

*For minimal back stress
and maximum ease of
movement*

I t is often assumed — wrongly — that proper posture requires mimicking the traditional military attention stance characterized by pulled-back shoulders, tucked-in chin and excessively arched lower back. Unlike this static, rigid configuration, posture is dynamic, and so requires continual adjustments. It incorporates the countless ways in which you align your spine and its supporting structures to allow common everyday positions such as sitting, standing, sleeping and carrying.

Good posture — keeping your spine aligned in a correct and comfortable position — demands careful balancing among the many bones, joints and muscles of the back. When the back is properly aligned, you will maximize the spaces between the 24 vertebrae along the spinal column, thus lengthening the spine and allowing the vertebrae to move easily in relation to one another. The advantage of this maximum spacing is that it avoids spinal compression, thus placing the least possible stress on your spine. Correct posture also allows you to maintain the desired configuration of the three curves in your back: the forward curves of the neck and lower back, and the backward curve of the middle spine.

Poor posture often leads to an exaggeration of the back's normal curves. In particular, swayback — a hyperlordosis, or excessive curvature, of the lower back — contributes significantly to back problems by pulling the vertebrae of the lower back out of alignment. The misalignment compresses the facet joints at the back of the vertebrae, causing them to wear down. Abnormal spinal alignment also places demands on the supporting ligaments and musculature of the back, forcing certain muscles to compensate, while others are underutilized as a result.

Not only is posture dynamic, it is interdependent, involving the head, shoulders, hips and legs as well as the spine itself. For example, an exaggerated curvature in one area of the back can lead to compensating misalignments elsewhere. Thus, if you have swayback, you very well might have hyperkyphosis, or a rounded upper back and shoulders, plus hyperlordosis in the neck. Likewise, improper lifting — using the back muscles themselves rather than the quadriceps muscles in the thighs — can strain the back extensors, thus reducing their effectiveness in spinal support. Because of this interdependence, many back-care specialists treat the whole body, including the neck, shoulders and hip joints.

There is a reciprocal relationship between posture and the supporting musculature of the back: Good muscle tone is necessary for proper posture, and proper posture enables your muscles to function appropriately. For example, strong abdominal muscles will allow you to maintain the optimum curve in your lower back, while weak abdominals permit the spine to curve forward, creating a hyperlordosis, which shortens the muscles of the back and compresses the vertebrae.

Improving the tone of the muscles that support your spine will help to reduce excess curvatures. However, good muscle tone does not in itself ensure good posture. Even if your muscle tone is adequate, poor habits like slumped sitting, stooped standing and rounded shoulders can develop over a period of years, frequently beginning in adolescence.

Retraining yourself to overcome bad posture can be a challenge. Because they are familiar, the positions you commonly assume for standing and sitting probably feel right. Therefore, edicts such as "sit up straight," or "pull your head back" are likely to elicit a temporary response at best. Some researchers believe that performing exercises aimed at improving your sense of what feels correct is the most effective approach to undoing bad habits.

The Alexander technique is one method that uses self-awareness to "teach" the entire spine and back to move with less stress and greater efficiency. Developed at the turn of the century by F.M. Alexander, the technique helps you replace dysfunctional movement habits with improved ones. In one study based on the Alexander technique, participants were first told to sit in their normal relaxed position. They

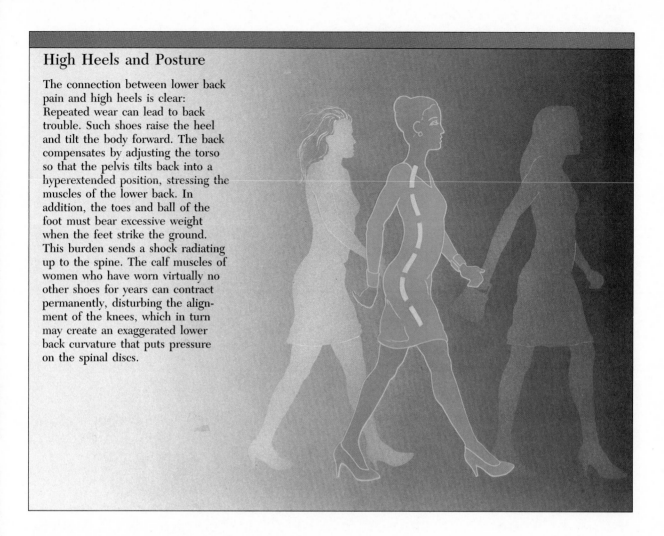

High Heels and Posture

The connection between lower back pain and high heels is clear: Repeated wear can lead to back trouble. Such shoes raise the heel and tilt the body forward. The back compensates by adjusting the torso so that the pelvis tilts back into a hyperextended position, stressing the muscles of the lower back. In addition, the toes and ball of the foot must bear excessive weight when the feet strike the ground. This burden sends a shock radiating up to the spine. The calf muscles of women who have worn virtually no other shoes for years can contract permanently, disturbing the alignment of the knees, which in turn may create an exaggerated lower back curvature that puts pressure on the spinal discs.

were then told to correct their sitting in two ways: First by simply being directed to sit up straight and second by being guided into an improved sitting alignment using Alexander principles. Neck muscle tension of participants increased sharply when they were told to sit up straight, but they experienced a decrease in muscular tension — coupled with the desired spine lengthening — when they used the Alexander instructions.

The Alexander-based exercises in this chapter are designed to train muscles during ordinary movement so that you will become familiar with good posture as you sit, stand and walk. Some exercises, like those in the sitting alignment routine on pages 80-81, demonstrate the different sensations that good and bad posture create. Others, such as the shoulder circles on page 86, tone the muscles associated with posture as they improve alignment. As you become familiar with how your back feels when you move through these positions, you will find it easy to discard your old postural habits and replace them with improved ones.

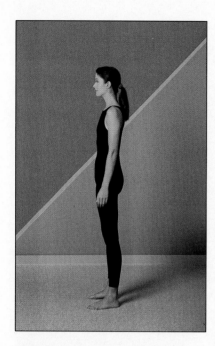

STANDING Stand with your feet spread slightly and your arms at your sides *(above)*. Tighten your abdominals as you raise your arms over your head in front of you *(right)*. Keep your arms shoulder-width apart. Return to the starting position. Perform four repetitions.

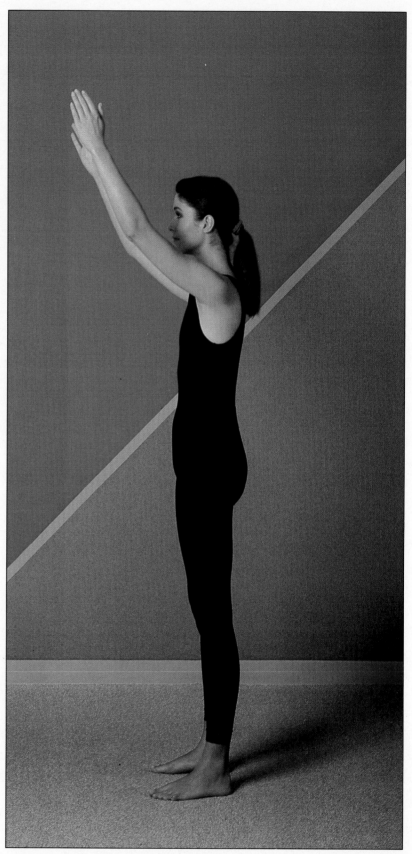

Aligning Your Spine

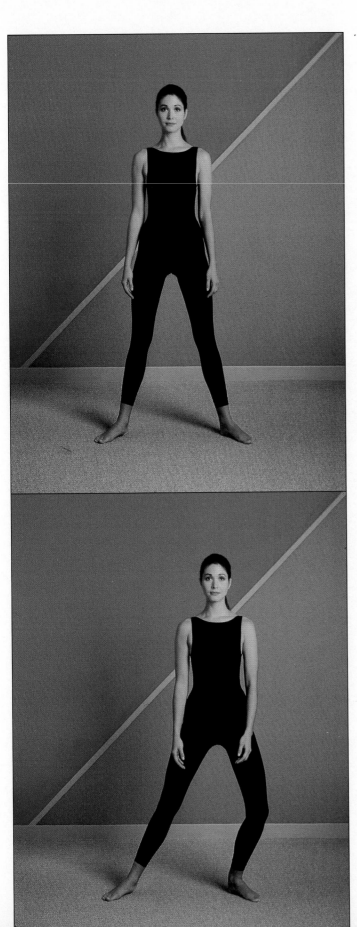

The basic principle behind the exercises on these two pages and the following 18 is to keep your spine aligned and elongated, achieving the maximum possible length from your neck to your coccyx. To visualize this while you perform the exercises, imagine a thread being pulled gently from the top of your head, drawing your spine upward as it positions the vertebrae on top of one another.

The exercises are not designed to be strenuous, but rather to encourage postural awareness and help you acquire habits that you can use in everyday activities. Thus, careful monitoring of your movements and exacting adjustments are more important than the number of repetitions or the speed of the execution. If possible, perform the exercises in front of a mirror so that you can observe the curvatures of your spine.

Practice the exercises daily. Doing so while imagining your spine in proper alignment will retrain your posture habits. Through the process of exercise combined with picturing your spine and observation, you can internalize new ways of moving so that you go through your daily activities with grace and efficiency.

STANDING Take a comfortably wide stance with your arms at your sides *(top)*. Bend your left knee, letting your torso move to the left. Keep your spine lengthened *(left)*. Straighten your knee; repeat to the right. Alternate sides 10 times.

Standing/2

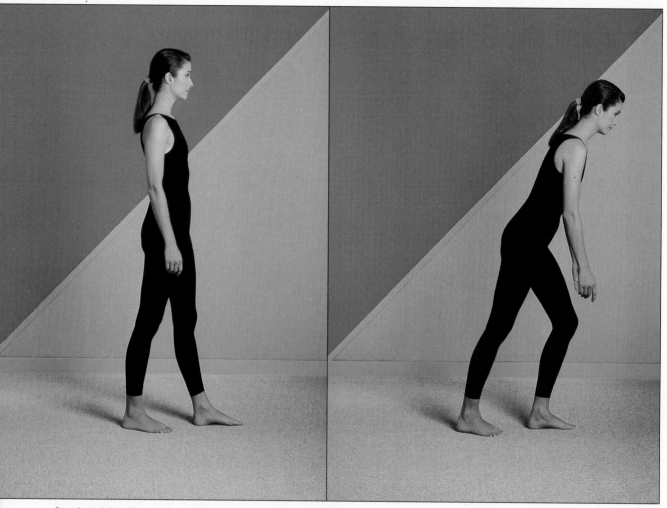

Stand straight with your feet slightly spread and your left foot in front of your right *(above)*. Lean forward, bending your left knee and keeping your back straight *(right)*. Straighten your leg and return to the starting position. Repeat five times; switch legs.

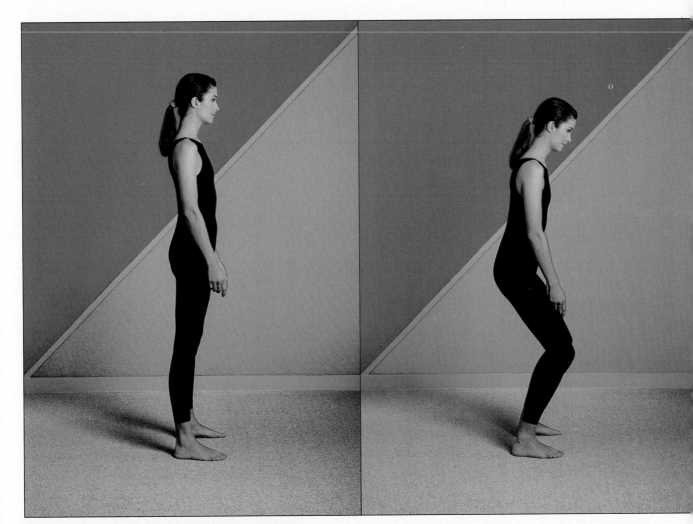

From a standing position with your feet shoulder-width apart
(above), bend both knees and lean forward *(right)*. Keep your
spine aligned and use your hips to tilt your torso forward. Keep
your arms relaxed; straighten your body. Repeat five times.

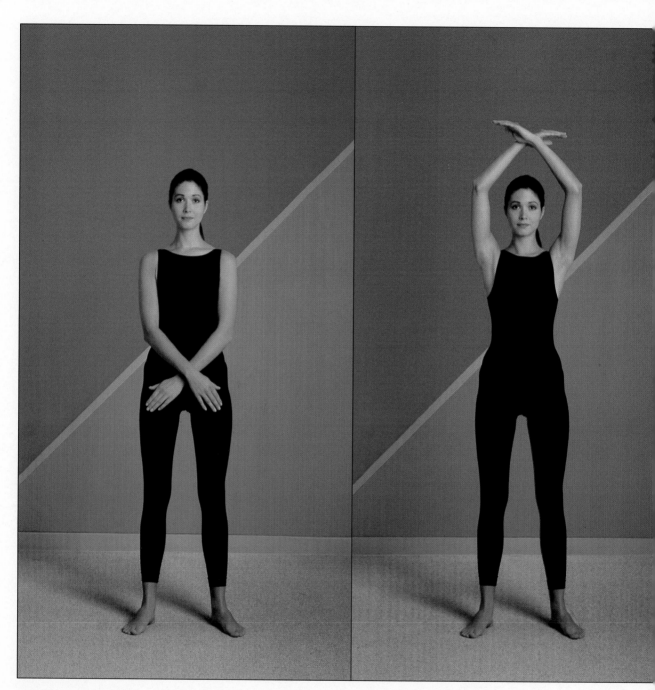

Standing/3

Stand with your feet shoulder-width apart and cross your arms in front of you *(above)*. Make large arm circles by slowly raising your crossed arms *(left center)*, then opening them up *(right center)* and bringing them down to your sides *(far right)*. Return to the starting position and repeat five times.

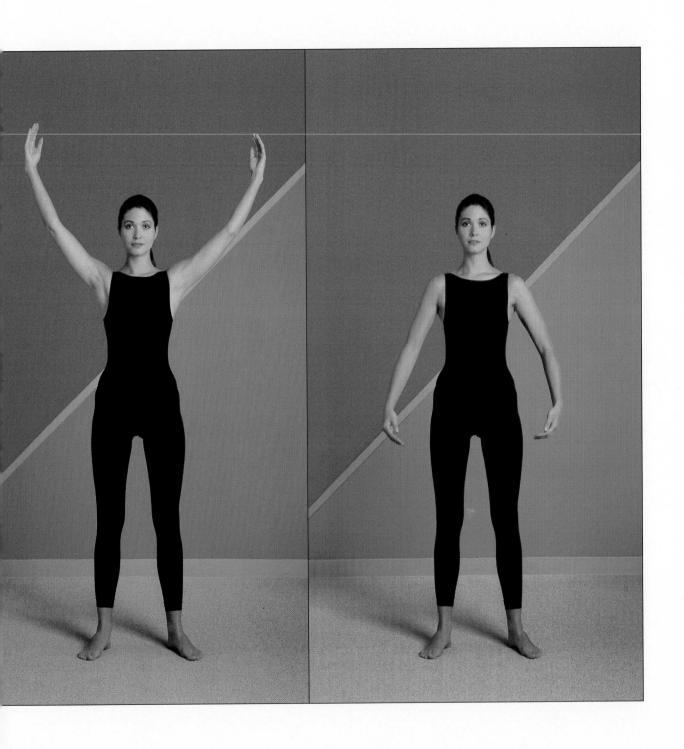

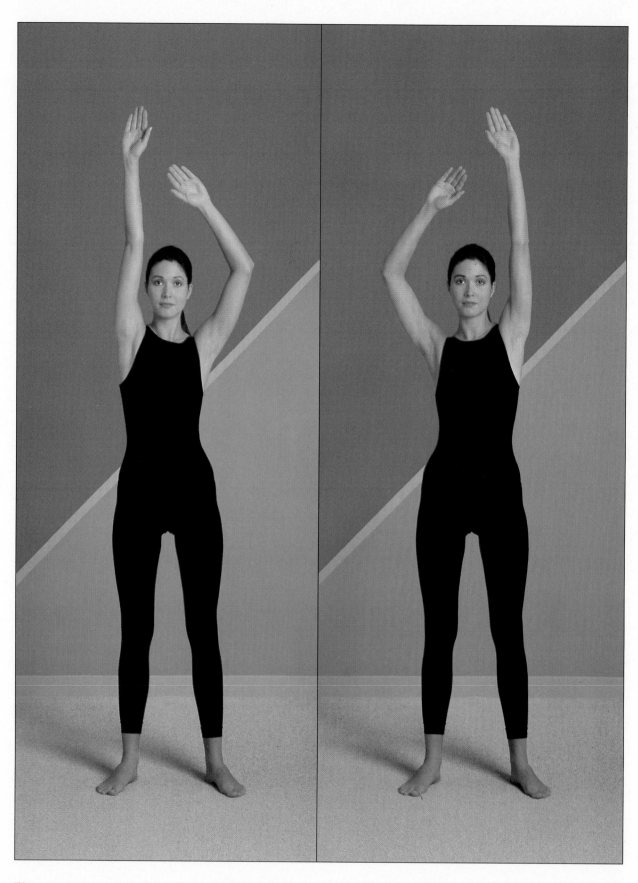

Standing/4

Raise your arms over your head, keeping them shoulder-width apart. Alternately reach with your right and then your left arm *(opposite)*. Tighten your abdominals as you reach. Alternate arms 10 times.

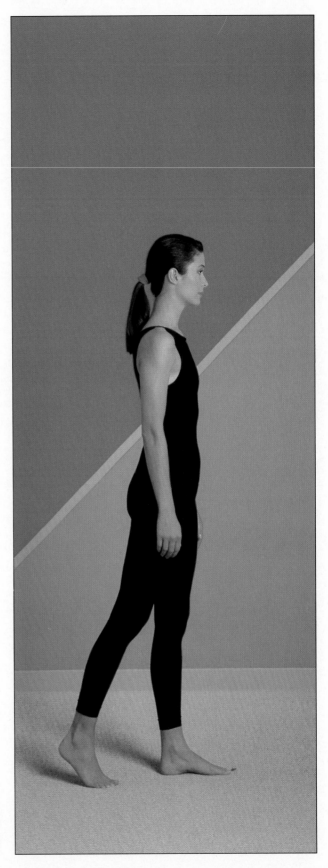

Walk for one minute, keeping your spine lengthened and your arms relaxed at your sides. Alternate tightening your abdominals for four steps and releasing them for the next four steps.

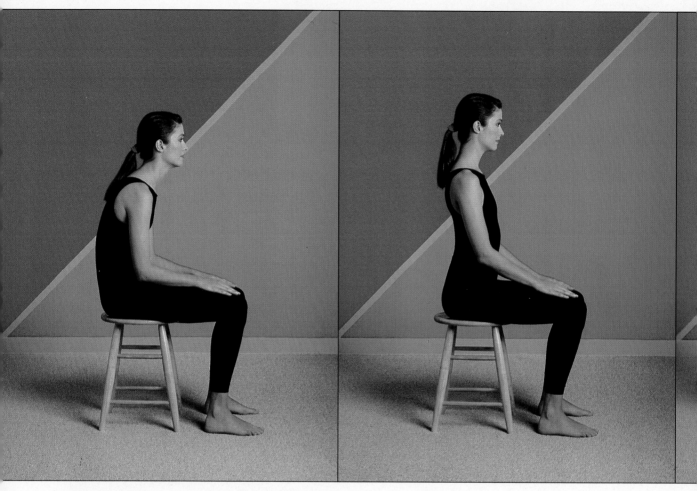

Sitting/1

Sit on a stool or a chair with your back unsupported. To find your correct body alignment, slouch forward *(above)*, then arch your lower back as much as possible *(center)*, then assume an upright position between these two extremes *(right)*. Repeat three times.

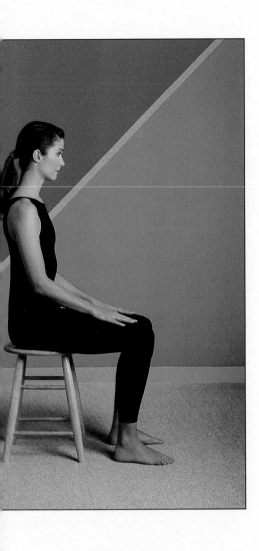

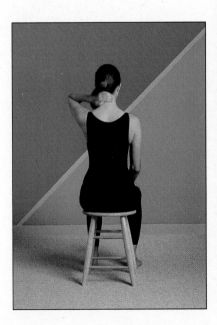

Place one hand loosely around the back of your neck. While looking straight ahead, gently bring your neck back toward your hand as you think of lengthening your neck and entire spine. Hold for a count of five; repeat three times.

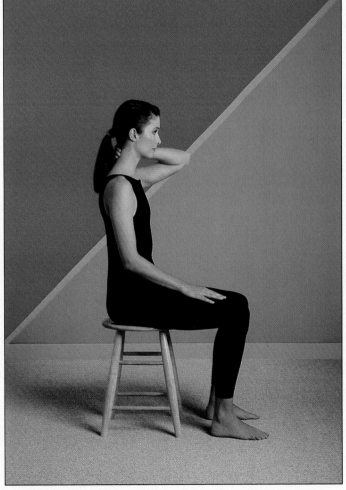

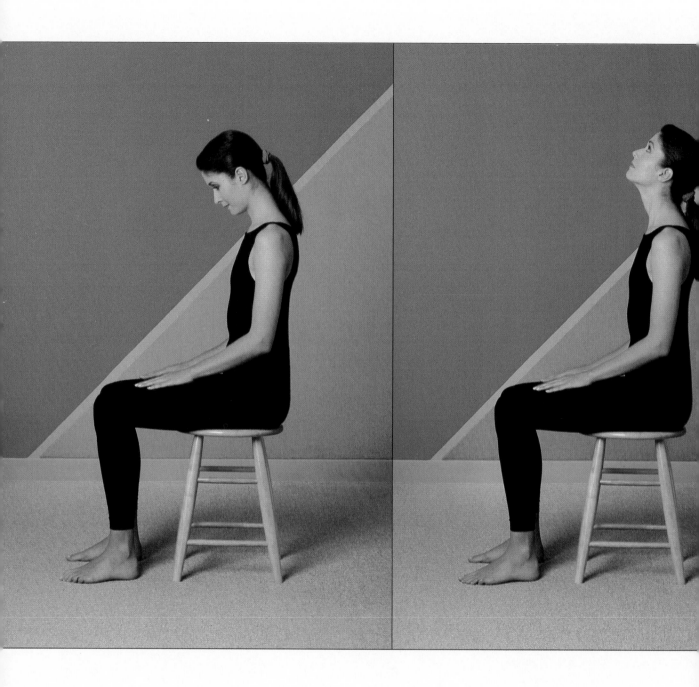

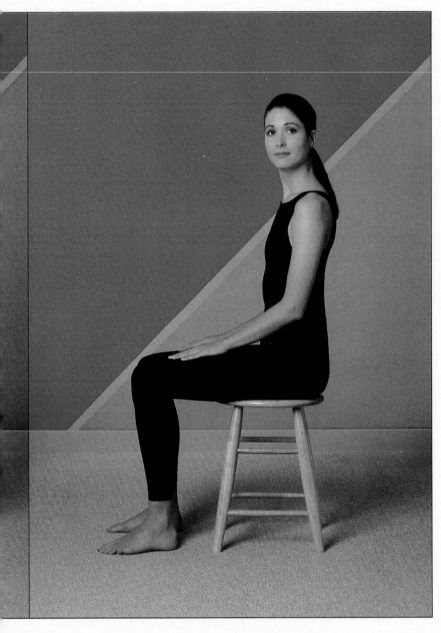

Sitting/2

Sit on a chair or stool with your feet flat on the floor, your hands resting on your lap and your back straight. Look down *(far left)*, look up *(center)*, then look to each side *(near left)*. Make sure to keep your spine lengthened as you move your head. Repeat five times.

Sitting/3

Clockwise from top left: Sit on a stool with your hands at your sides. Raise your arms and extend them out to the sides, keeping your shoulders even. Raise your arms over your head and bend your elbows so that your forearms rest lightly on your head. Raise your arms back up, out and down to return to the starting position, as you lengthen your head and spine. Repeat three times.

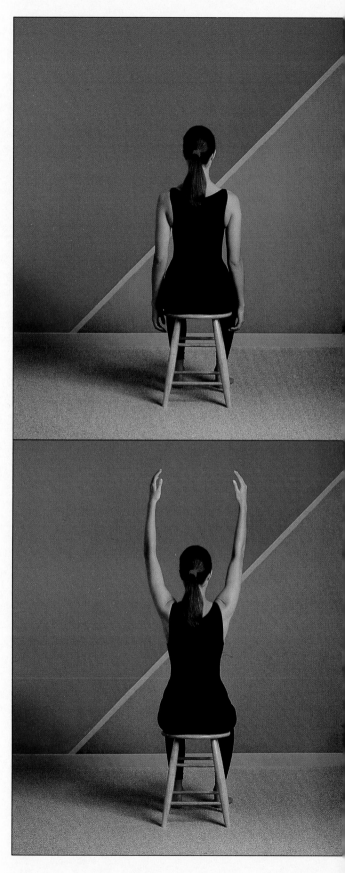

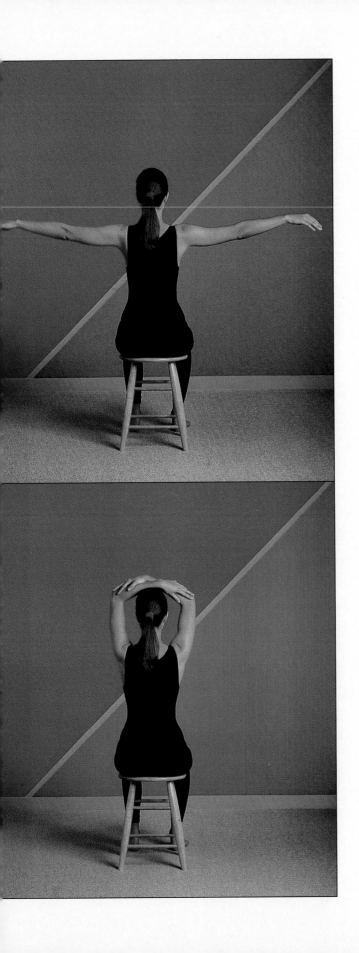

Sitting/4

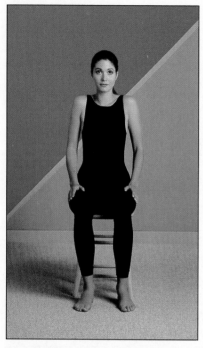

From a sitting position, circle your shoulders by bringing them up *(above)*, back *(right)*, down and forward. Keep your spine lengthened. Repeat five times.

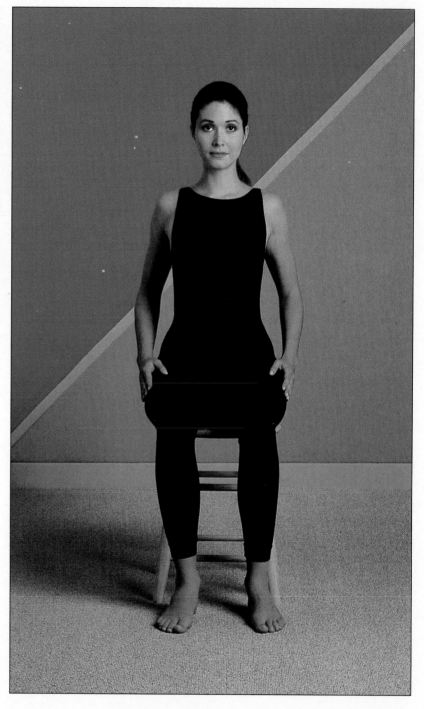

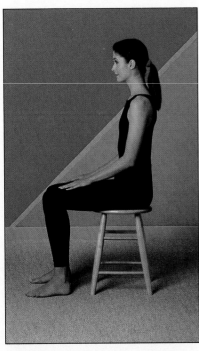

Sit on a chair or stool with your spine
lengthened and your feet flat on the floor
in front of you *(above)*. Lean forward,
keeping your spine aligned *(right)*. Return
and repeat five times.

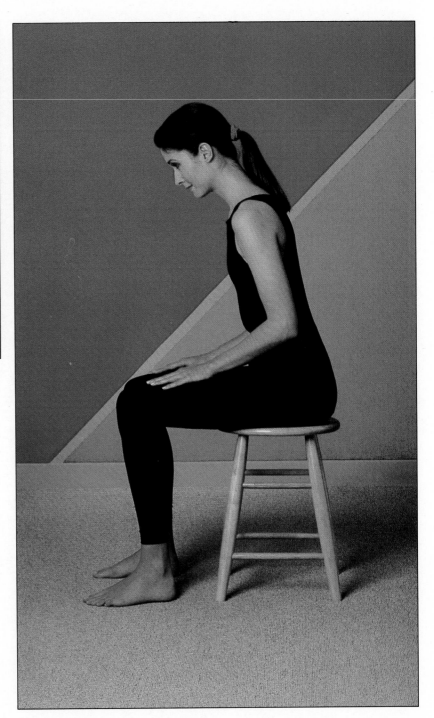

Sitting/5

Sit erect on a chair or stool with your spine elongated and your hands resting lightly on your thighs. Gently tighten your abdominals five times.

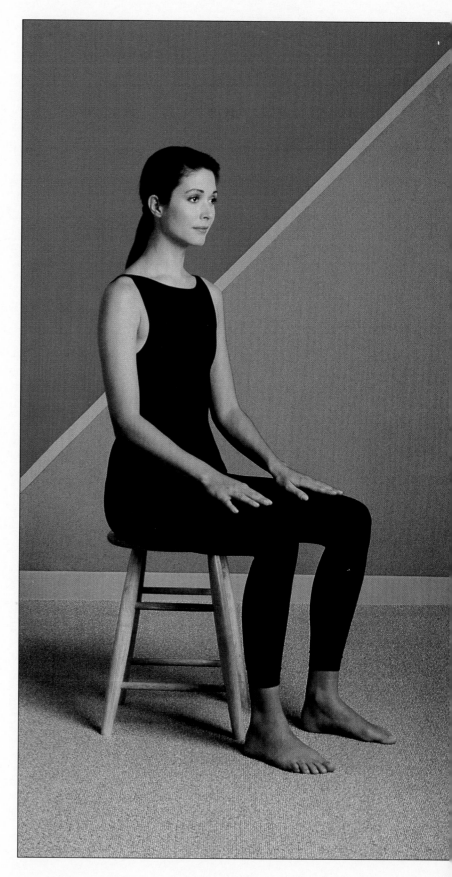

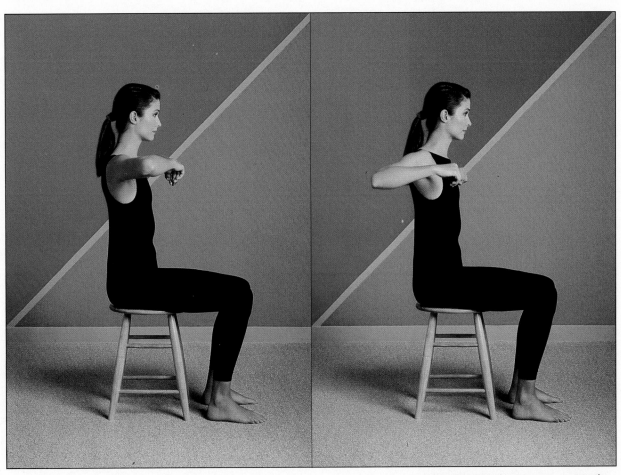

While seated, raise your arms out to the side to shoulder height, with your elbows bent *(left)*. Pull your shoulders back five times, drawing your shoulder blades together *(above);* lower your arms. Repeat three times.

Lying Down

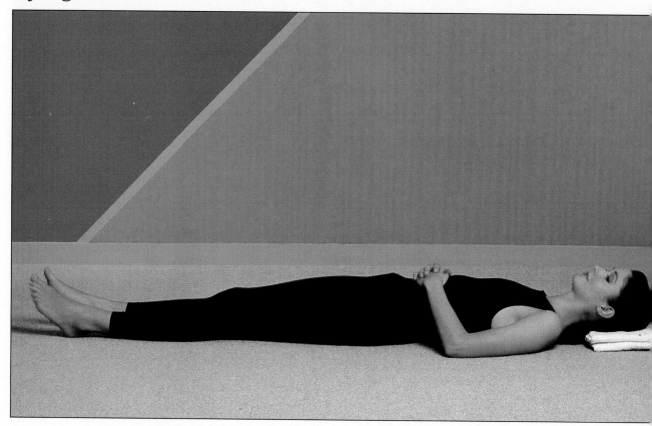

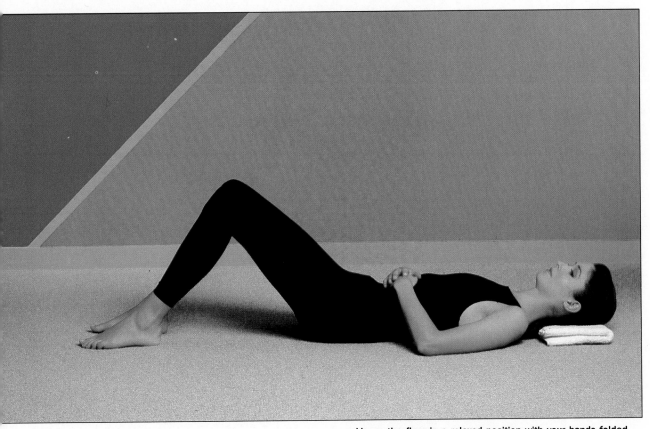

Lie on the floor in a relaxed position with your hands folded over your abdomen *(opposite)*. Place a small pillow or folded towel under your head to keep your neck aligned. Bend your legs so that your feet lie flat on the floor *(above)*. Keeping your hips in place, stretch your spine by flattening your lower back against the floor, and then moving your shoulders and head along the floor away from your hips. Maintaining this alignment, rest for a count of 10 or longer.

Breathing Techniques

All the back muscles that attach to the ribs or lie below them are affected by breathing. Proper breathing allows this musculature to relax and keeps it well supplied with oxygen. Indeed, breathing correctly helps promote relaxation and can even reduce back problems by breaking the cycle of tension and pain.

Improving your posture by performing such exercises as shown on the preceding 18 pages can ease your breathing. When you reduce spinal compression, you provide more room for your muscles to expand and contract freely. This is especially important for the diaphragm, the primary muscle involved in breathing. This muscle is attached to the lower ribs as well as to some of the vertebrae of the spine. Overtightening the muscles of the chest and neck will interfere with correct breathing. In contrast, a well-balanced spine allows you to use your diaphragm and other muscles to breathe correctly.

You can tell if you are breathing properly by the way your abdomen and rib cage move: On inhalation, they should expand, and on exhalation, they move back inward. The two exercises shown here will help you evaluate your breathing and concentrate on improving it.

Sit up straight in a chair. Place your hands on either side of your rib cage, with your thumbs toward your back. Breathe naturally. Keep your spine lengthened as you feel your ribs move in and out with each breath.

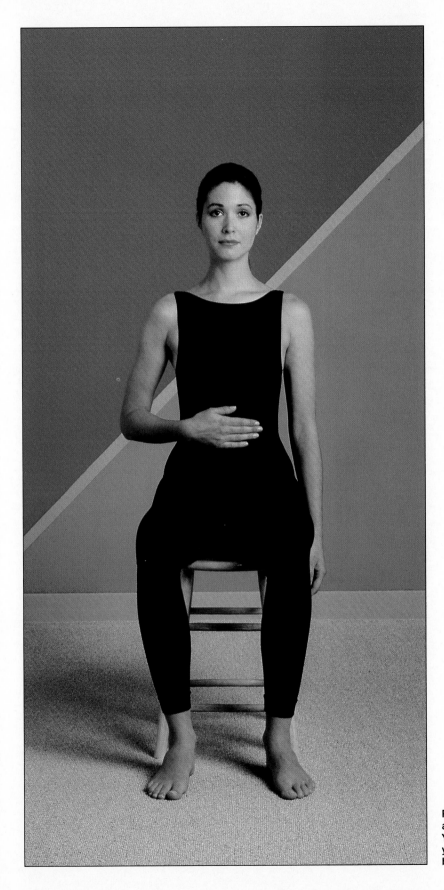

Place one hand at the center of your abdomen at waist level. Breathe naturally. You should feel your abdomen expand as you breathe in and move inward as you breathe out.

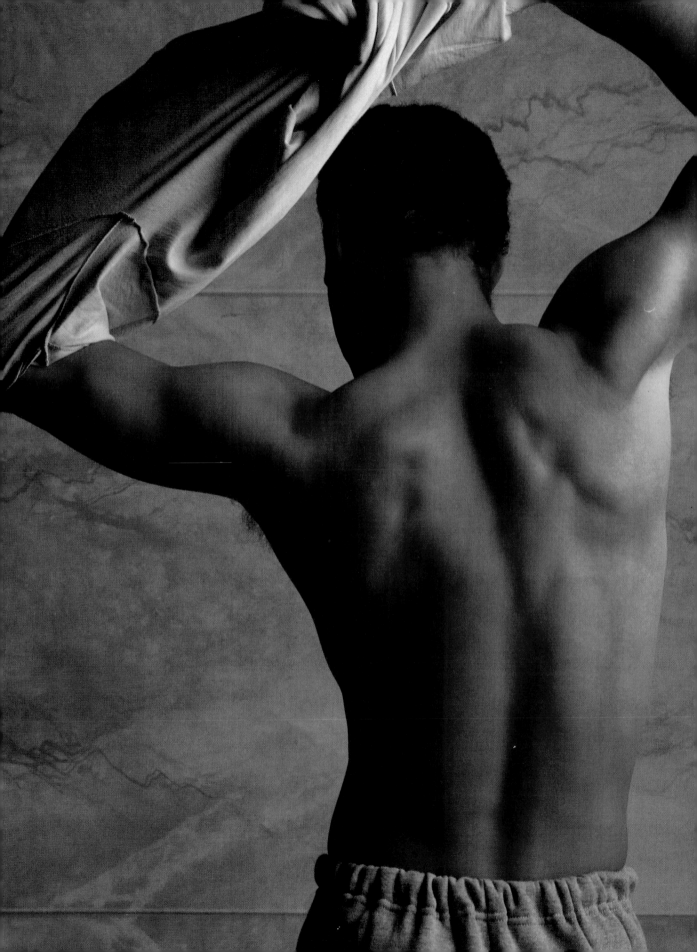

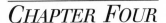

CHAPTER FOUR

Day-to-Day Back Care

Techniques for protecting your back in everyday situations

Good posture and well-toned muscles provide the foundation for a fit back, but these two basic elements of back care are effective only if you integrate them into the performance of daily activities like driving a car, lifting an infant, carrying a suitcase and other maneuvers that can become sources of back strain. This chapter will show you efficient ways of standing, sitting and moving that you can apply to almost any situation that involves your back.

The spine's flexibility allows you to combine considerable mobility with strength. When done properly, any normal movement is within the spine's range and can be performed without strain. Unfortunately, the spine is often used incorrectly. In particular, the waist is commonly used as a hinge joint between the lower and the upper body, forcing it to work like a knee or an elbow. But the waist is not a joint, and trying to use it as one can strain or overstretch the muscles and ligaments of the lower back.

For bending movements, the hips allow the torso — pelvis and spine — to move forward as a unit. Bending, leaning and lifting should all be accomplished with the hips rather than the waist. This will allow you to use the muscles of the torso correctly to maintain vertebral alignment.

Lifting offers one of the best examples of the importance of moving properly. No other common maneuver places as much stress on the lower back as picking up an object from the floor with your knees straight and your torso bent at the waist. The bent-knee technique, shown on pages 104-105, illustrates the right way to lift: flexing your hips and bending your knees, using the quadriceps muscles in the front of the thigh for power and concentrating on upper body alignment. Your abdominals and the large muscles of the thigh share the burden of lowering and lifting, relieving the back muscles and the spine itself of the load.

Another common activity that poses risks to the lower back is sitting. In fact, sitting creates more strain than walking, standing or lying down, and its stresses account largely for the high incidence of lower back pain among office workers. Physicians report that many years spent sitting in office jobs can cause a condition known as fibrous contracture, characterized by a shortening of the muscles in the back and a resulting loss of elasticity. This condition of overall inflexibility often makes it difficult and even painful for the sufferer to bend forward.

One of the best ways to ease the stress of sitting is to find a good chair. A soft, overstuffed sofa can be just as hard on the back as a backless stool or poorly designed desk chair — none of them provides adequate lower back support. When you choose a chair, find one with a firm, padded, adjustable back that can tilt backward about 10 degrees. Its seat should support your thighs at a 90-degree angle to your lower legs, or your knees can be slightly higher than your hips. If you do not have a suitable chair, maintaining proper posture and using cushions for lumbar support can still help overcome the strain of prolonged sitting (see pages 108-109). Interrupting periods of sitting with stretching, walking or simply shifting positions is also recommended to prevent your back from becoming stiff and inflexible. Examples of good chairs, lumbar pillows and other items designed for the back appear on pages 98-99.

Some people react to potential back problems by overprotecting themselves and avoiding activities — including sports and sex — that they fear might trigger back pain. In fact, physical activity can actually benefit the back, as long as the activity is carefully chosen (see box at right). You do not have to forgo sex unless you have acute back pain and muscle spasm; otherwise, you need only take care to use positions for intercourse that are easy on your back. Many back specialists recommend lying on your side, either facing your partner or lying back to front. Alternately, if the partner with the back problem is on top during sex, he or she will be more comfortable if the other person

Choosing a Sport

Having a back problem is no reason to avoid sports, but you should follow certain guidelines in deciding which sport or exercise routines to engage in. The most important rule is to maintain proper conditioning of the back's supporting muscles. Strong, flexible muscles are the best guarantee of staying injury-free. Here are other tips to keep in mind:

◆ The exercises most highly recommended for people with back problems are swimming (except for the butterfly and breaststroke, which require arching your back), walking, cross-country skiing and cycling (as long as you use an upright posture). These sports are also excellent cardiovascular conditioners, so that you will build endurance as you improve your back muscles.

◆ In the poorly conditioned individual, racquet sports, golf and other activities that involve twisting the torso can imperil the back. Bowling can also pose a risk because it requires lifting a heavy weight. Besides straining the back muscles, a sudden twist can cause a ruptured disc if the movement is too abrupt. Sports-medicine specialists have noted, however, that such injuries tend to occur because of incorrect techniques or insufficient warm-ups, not because they are intrinsic to any sport.

◆ Certain other exercise movements can put you at risk of back pain. Running and aerobic dance can be jarring to the back, but you can minimize the stress by wearing proper shoes and working out on a surface resilient enough to cushion the shock. If you are performing routines to improve muscle tone, be sure to avoid straight-leg sit-ups and bilateral leg-lifts, which can irritate the spinal nerves. If you lift weights, take care not to overarch your back. It is also wise to wear a lifting belt and to work with a spotter.

is propped up with extra cushions. This facilitates a bent-knee position for the partner on top, because it tilts the pelvis forward to minimize lower back stress.

The techniques described in the following 18 pages will help you put into practice the postural and muscular development outlined in the previous chapters. Indeed, the practical movement applications demonstrated in this chapter are really extensions of the preceding routines. Understanding these concepts and retraining your body to these new ways of moving will go a long way toward maintaining a healthy back.

The chapter concludes with trigger point and massage sequences that you and your partner can use. Both trigger point and massage therapy are commonly used in the physical rehabilitation of back patients. However, they serve important preventive functions as well. In its most basic form, trigger point therapy entails a simple finger-pressure technique that can pinpoint and alleviate specific problems that may contribute to back pain. Likewise, massage is a hands-on therapy that eases overall muscle tension in your back. Using both techniques as a regular part of your back-care regimen is a pleasant way to protect your back from the strain it can undergo during the course of a day.

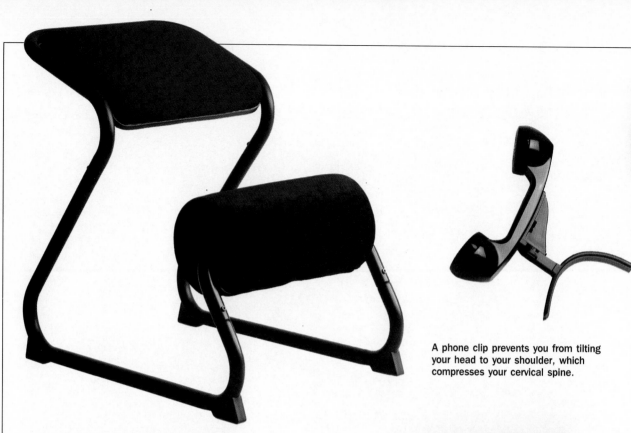

A phone clip prevents you from tilting your head to your shoulder, which compresses your cervical spine.

A kneeling chair, by putting the weight of your body on your knees, encourages your torso to maintain balance and alignment.

Lumbar cushions can provide the lower back support that a chair, couch or car seat may lack.

Back Aids

Having the proper equipment and furniture can facilitate back care, as well as prevent back pain or injury. There is no dearth of products designed to benefit your back; however, all such items are user-specific. Because what is comfortable for someone else might be irritating to your back, it is important to try out anything you intend to purchase, particularly chairs and mattresses. Similarly, although back-supporting equipment and furniture comes in a wide range of prices, cost is not necessarily a true indicator of quality or appropriateness.

A sampling of chairs and accessories intended to provide maximum support and to relieve muscular tension in the back area appears on these two pages.

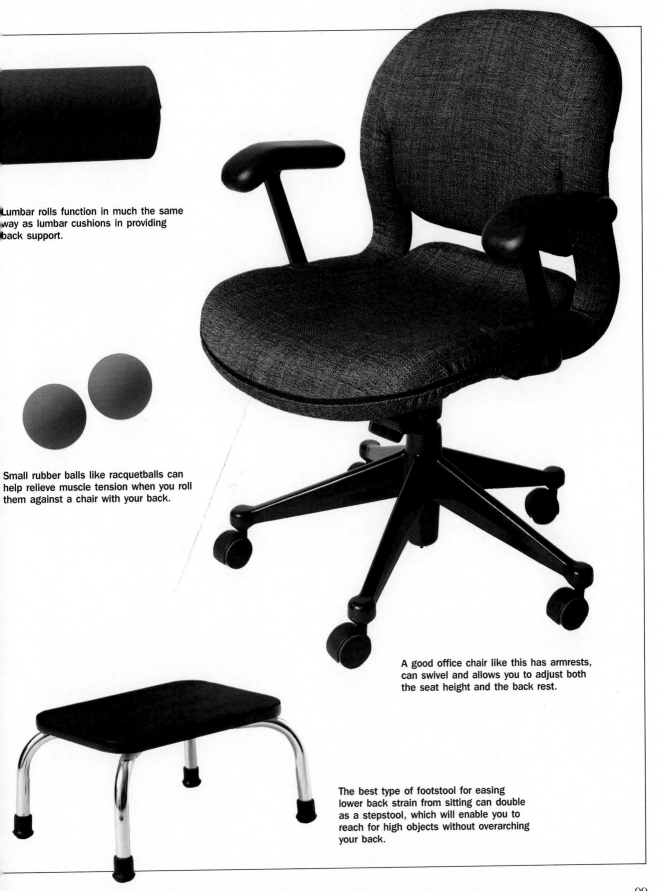

Lumbar rolls function in much the same way as lumbar cushions in providing back support.

Small rubber balls like racquetballs can help relieve muscle tension when you roll them against a chair with your back.

A good office chair like this has armrests, can swivel and allows you to adjust both the seat height and the back rest.

The best type of footstool for easing lower back strain from sitting can double as a stepstool, which will enable you to reach for high objects without overarching your back.

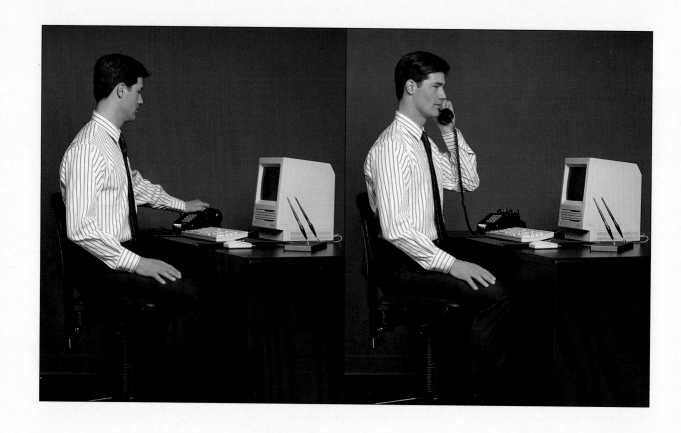

In the Office

Position your office phone on your left side if you are right-handed, and vice versa . It should be less than an arm's length away from your usual sitting position. As you reach for the receiver, keep your back resting against your chair and your torso aligned *(above left)*. Bring the phone all the way up to your ear, keeping your head erect as you talk *(above right)* or use a phone clip, as shown on the preceding page.

Adapting your office environment to accommodate your back can greatly reduce the stress of a sedentary job. Choosing the proper furniture, such as the chairs shown on the preceding two pages, is essential. It is crucial that whatever furniture you use should be adjusted to your body proportions. The curve in the back of your chair should conform to your lumbar curve, and the chair seat should be set so that your knees are at least as high as your hips when your feet rest on the floor. The height of your desktop should be slightly above your waist when you are seated.

Frequent telephone use can pose some problems, especially if you are writing or reaching for something while holding the receiver. The right body mechanics, as shown above and at right, help you avoid unnecessary twisting in such situations. In addition, you should place the phone in an accessible spot so that you can reach anything you may need while you are talking. The proper placement and use of other equipment, like computers, typewriters and adding machines, can also ease potential back strain. If you are using a video display terminal, position it so that you need move only your eyes when looking from the keyboard to the terminal, allowing your head to remain still.

Take frequent breaks from sitting. Simply standing or taking a short walk will help release tension and avoid flexibility problems, as will performing the seated stretches shown on pages 66-67.

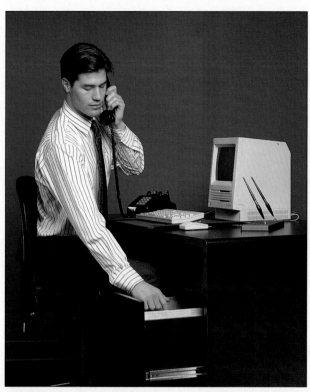

When reaching for something while you are on the phone, do not simply lean toward the object, but rotate your entire upper torso and bend forward from the hips *(above)*.

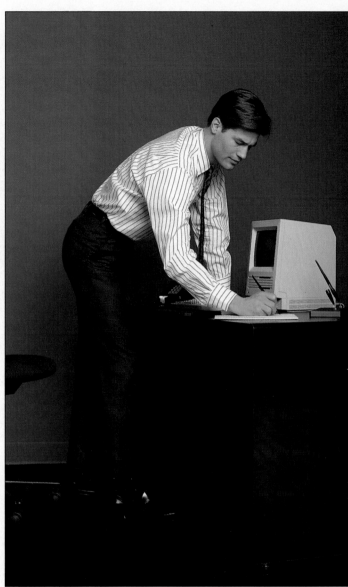

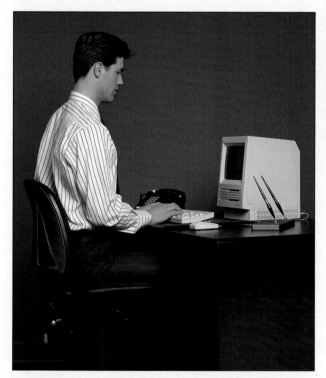

A desktop keyboard should be positioned directly in front of you. Rest your back against your chair and keep your arms at your sides with your elbows slightly bent. Use your wrists and hands *(above)*.

To lean over a desk and write from a standing position, stand with your feet shoulder-width apart in a lunge position. Rather than simply bending from the waist, lower your entire body by bending your knees and flexing at the hips *(above)*.

Daily Activity

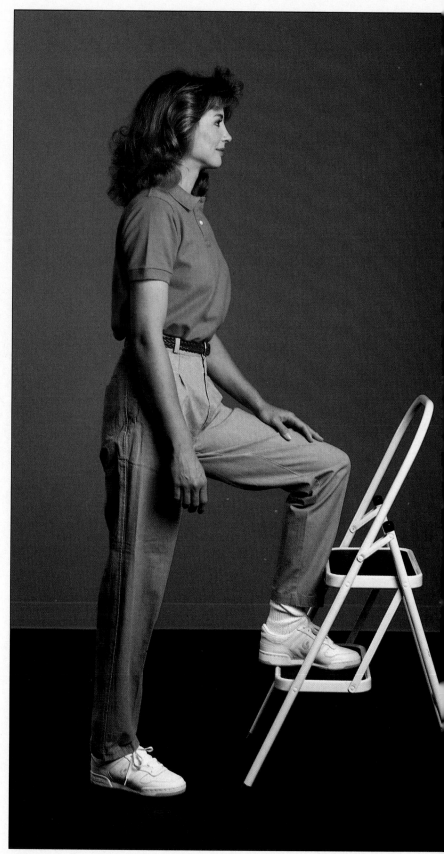

Using your back appropriately in everyday activities simply requires an awareness of how you move and, when necessary, making adjustments. For example, with many activities, haphazard movements can exaggerate the curve of the lower back, leading to back fatigue and possible injury. Such simple adjustments as bending your knees or using a stool can straighten the lower back, making it less prone to injury.

Virtually all the activities you perform — from carrying a briefcase to doing housework to reading in bed — utilize six basic movements: sitting, standing, reclining, lifting, bending and reaching. Guidelines for these six are outlined here and on the following 12 pages; each basic movement is followed by several illustrated applications. This page, for example, shows the correct technique for standing. The opposite page illustrates how to stand while cooking, putting on makeup or shaving, and brushing your teeth.

STANDING: When you stand for more than a few minutes, your vertebrae tend to sink down on themselves, which can make your lower back arch excessively. To avoid this, place one foot on a stool, book or any other similar object. Having one leg higher than the other will flatten the spinal curve.

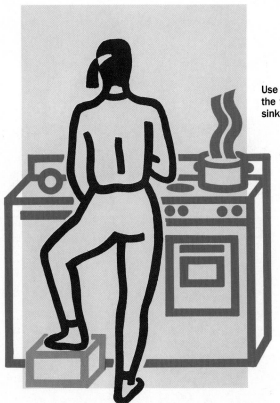

Use a stool or other footrest in the kitchen for the times you spend standing at the stove, sink or countertop.

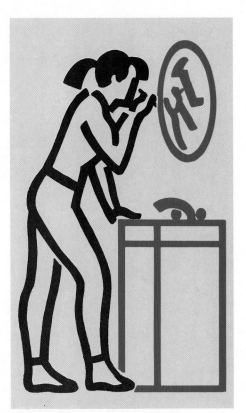

When leaning toward a mirror to apply makeup or to shave, stand in a lunging position and bend from the hips, keeping your back straight.

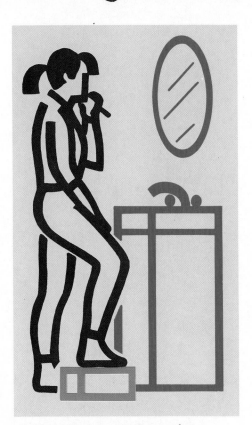

When brushing your teeth, place one foot on a stool. Bend forward from the hips when leaning over the sink.

Lifting

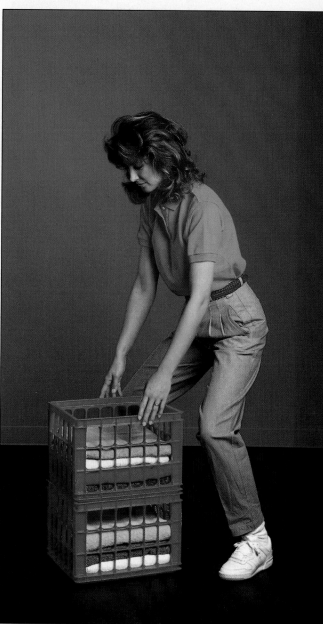

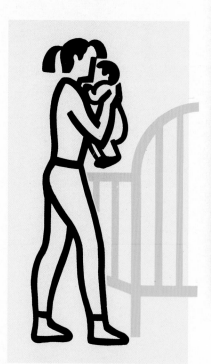

To lean over and lift, as when picking up a baby, assume a lunging position and bend from the hips *(top)*. Bring the baby close to you; then straighten up *(above)*.

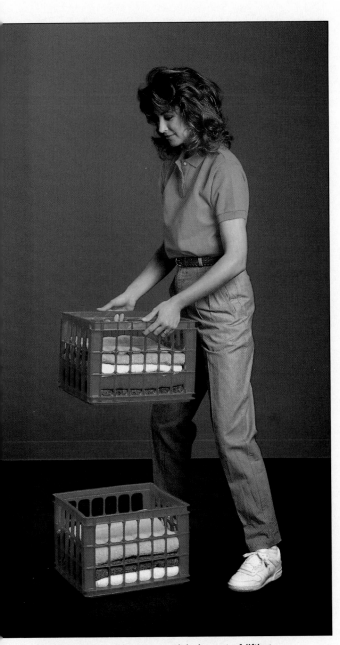

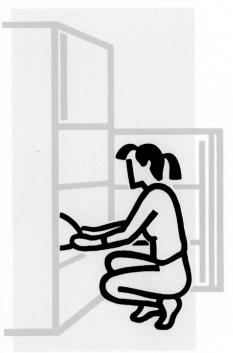

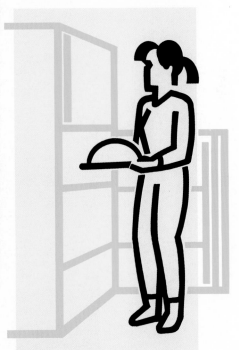

Proper positioning is an essential element of lifting. Stand close to the object you intend to lift and provide a broad base of support by spreading your feet wide on either side of it. Lower yourself by bending your knees, keeping your back aligned *(above left)*. Hold the object close to you as you straighten your legs to return to a standing position *(above)*.

To lift and twist, squat *(top)* and pull the item to you. Keep your knees and hips slightly bent as you turn and then rise *(above)*.

Carrying

Centering the load makes carrying easier. Keep your feet apart for a wide base and bend your knees slightly. Hold the object close to your torso so it can be supported by your body as well as your arms.

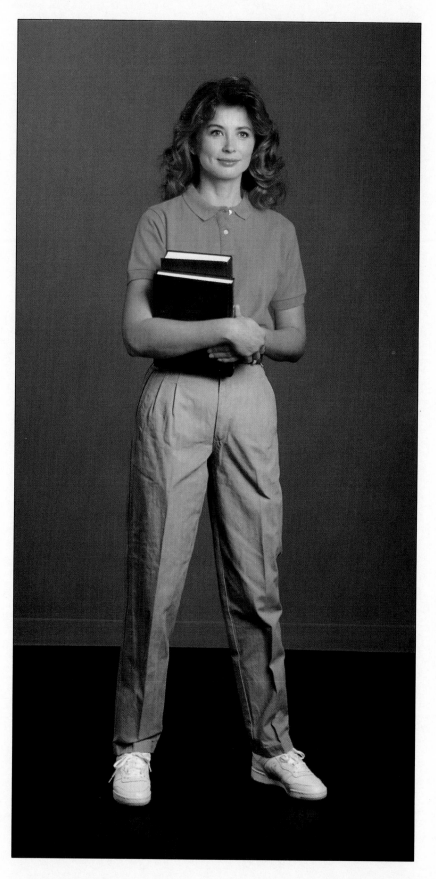

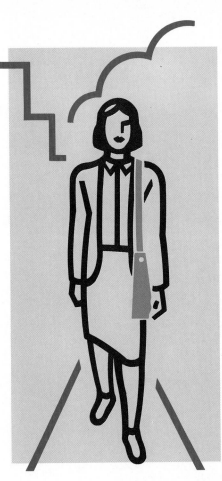

A briefcase with a shoulder strap helps spread the burden of weight to the upper torso. Adjust the strap length so you can put a hand underneath the briefcase to provide additional support. Switch sides periodically to relieve the weight.

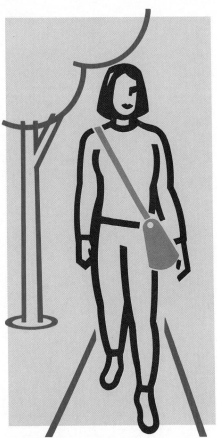

Distribute the weight of a pocketbook evenly on both sides of your body by carrying it with the strap across your chest. Place one hand underneath and hold it for extra support.

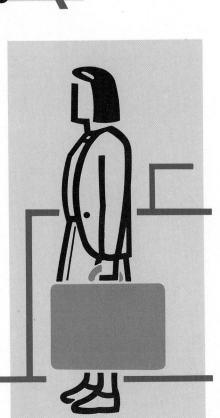

When you carry luggage, it is best to divide the weight evenly between two small suitcases. Otherwise, when carrying one large item, try to keep your shoulders level and provide a broad base with your feet. Alternate sides frequently.

Sitting

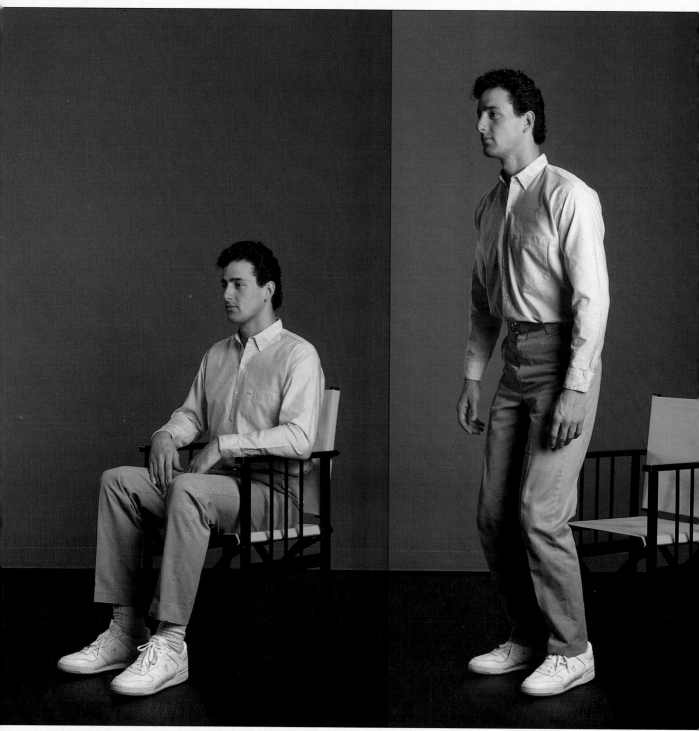

Sit all the way against the back of your chair. If the chair has arms, lean your arms on them for support *(above)*. To stand up, move to the edge of your chair and lean forward from your hips. Lead yourself out of the chair with your head, keeping your entire torso aligned *(above right)*.

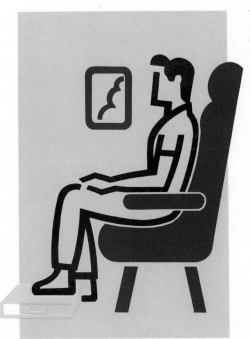

When traveling by plane or train, prop one foot on a piece of luggage. Alternate feet every 10-15 minutes to reduce lumbar compression.

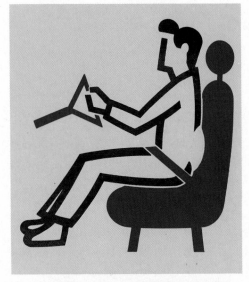

Position your car seat so that your elbows are bent when you grasp the steering wheel and your knees are slightly bent when reaching the floor pedals. Support your lower back with a small pillow or lumbar cushion to keep your torso alignment almost vertical.

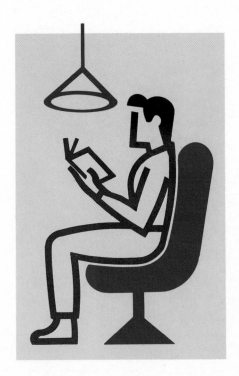

To read while seated, hold the book up at about chest level; avoid slumping forward. If your arms become tired, place a pillow on your lap to support the book.

Bending

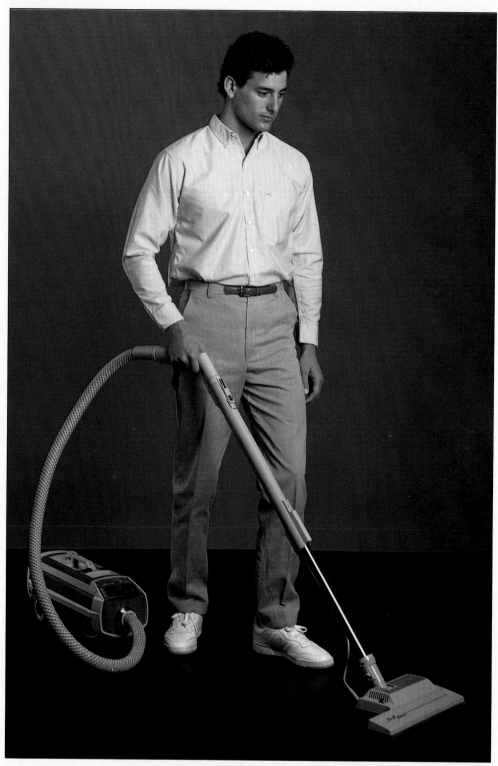

For house and yard work that requires bending and leaning, let your legs perform the majority of the work. When vacuuming, for example, stand with your feet shoulder-width apart. Place one foot in front of the other and move back and forth by shifting your weight from foot to foot. Bend from the hips to lower your torso.

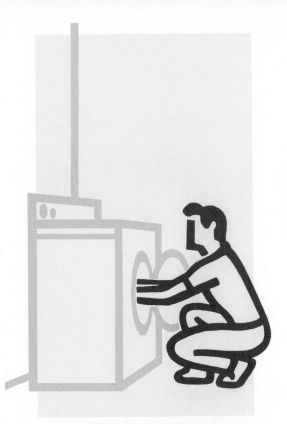

To reach into a dryer or dishwasher, lower your whole upper body by bending your knees and squatting.

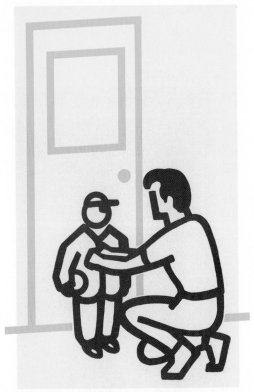

Use the same method as at left to button a child's coat. You can rest one knee on the floor for more support.

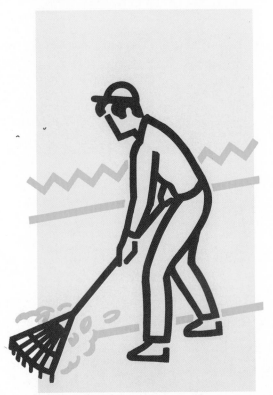

Use your feet as a broad base when raking. Reach down and forward by flexing your hips, keeping your spine aligned.

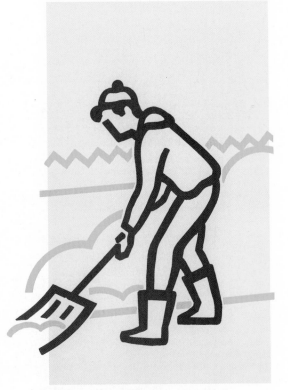

Place your hands well apart on a snow shovel to increase leverage. Bend at the hips to align your torso.

In Bed

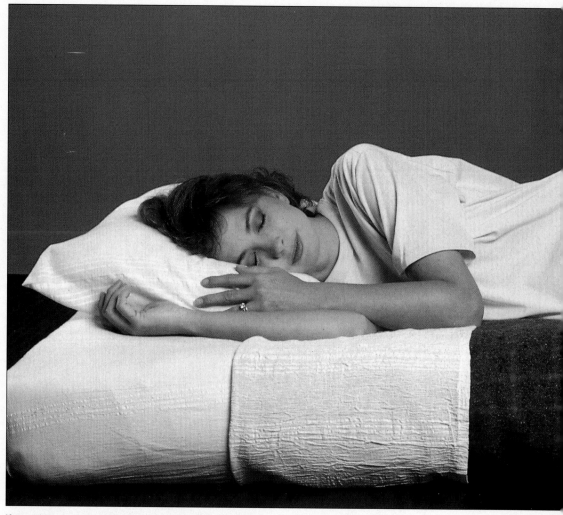

If you sleep on your side, place a semifirm, good-size pillow beneath your head and neck. Bend your knees and bring them up toward your chest. Place another pillow between your thighs and knees to reduce the pull exerted on your lower back by the upper legs.

Lying on your stomach is the worst position for your back, because it encourages arching of the lower back. If you must use this position, place a large pillow underneath your abdomen and bend one knee, bringing it up to the pillow. Do not use a pillow for your head.

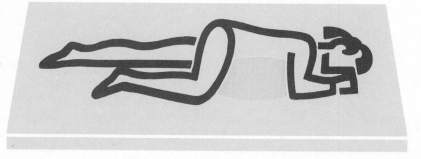

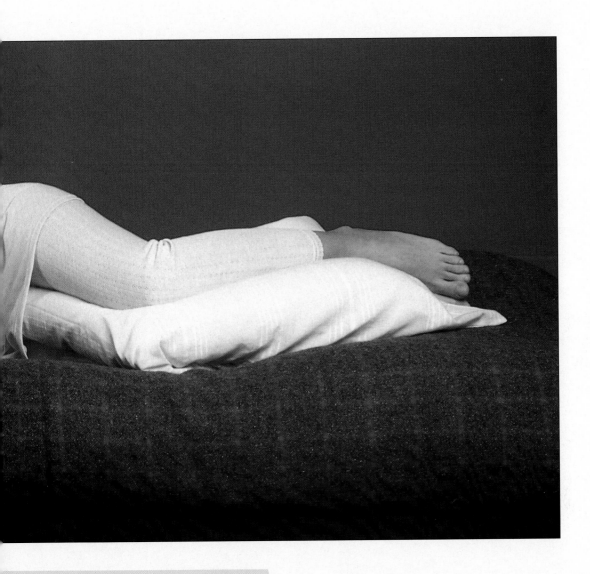

When sleeping on your back, place one or two good-size pillows under your knees to reduce the curve in your lower back. Your head and neck should be supported by another pillow.

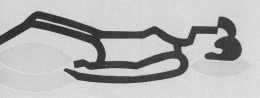

To read sitting up in bed, place one pillow lengthwise against the bedboard, another widthwise at the small of your back. Keep your knees bent by placing another pillow beneath them.

113

Reaching

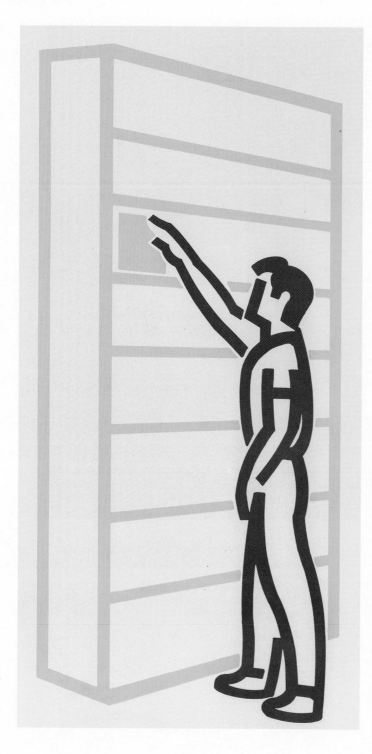

To reach for something placed above your head, stand within arm's length of the object in a lunge. The object should be low enough to reach without arching your lower back *(left)*. Otherwise, stand on a stool to avoid overextending your arm and back *(below)*.

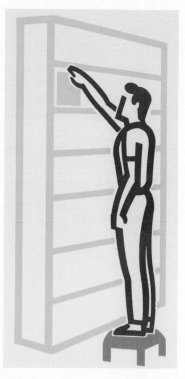

Socks and Shoes

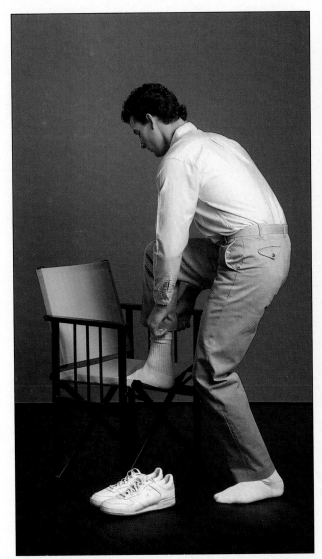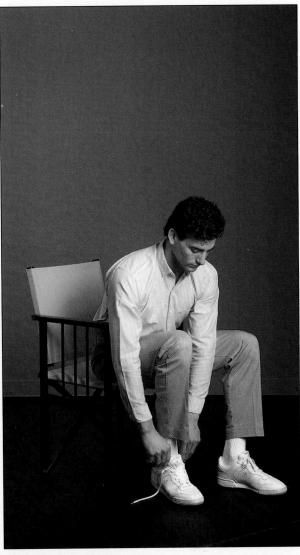

Because of the bending involved, people with back trouble frequently have problems getting dressed or undressed, particularly when reaching to their lower legs. To put on socks, raise one foot onto a chair or bed. Bend your other knee and lean forward from your hips, keeping your spine and neck aligned *(above)*. Switch legs and repeat. Sit down and bend forward from the hips to put your shoes on or take them off *(right)*.

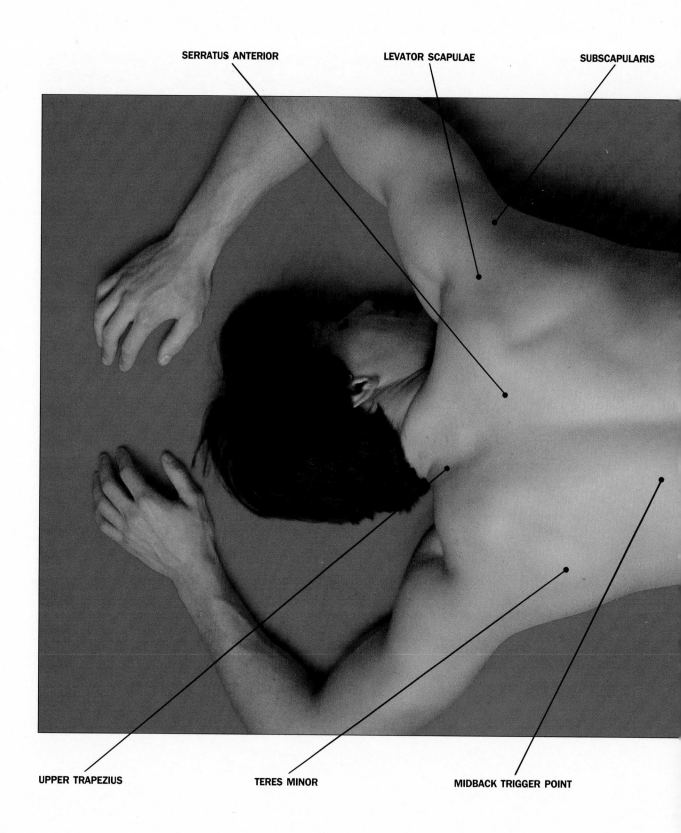

SERRATUS ANTERIOR

LEVATOR SCAPULAE

SUBSCAPULARIS

UPPER TRAPEZIUS

TERES MINOR

MIDBACK TRIGGER POINT

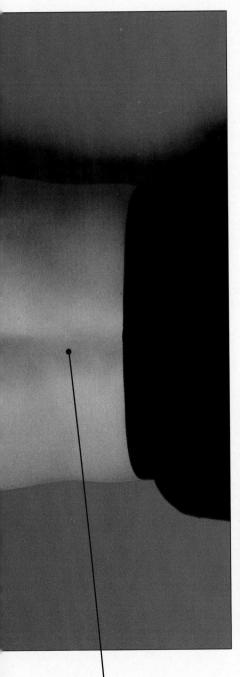

Trigger Points

One way to alleviate back pain is to treat trigger points, specific locations deep within a muscle in which by-products of exertion not flushed out by the circulatory system can collect. Stress or trauma can cause trigger points to become painful. In addition, poor posture as well as repetitive movements that lead to chronic muscle pain can irritate trigger points.

With the help of a friend, you can treat your trigger points both to prevent back-muscle tension and to relieve existing pain. Use the guide at left to find which trigger points correspond to potentially troublesome muscles. Because of lo-calized muscle tension and spasm, many trigger points feel like small nodules, which will help guide you and your partner to them.

Pressure on trigger points may feel uncomfortable but should not produce acute pain. In fact, you should feel relief immediately after a trigger point treatment. If a trigger point is especially sensitive, ask your partner to exert less pressure on it. Coordinating your partner's pressure with your breathing can also lessen pain: Your partner should exert pressure when you exhale and light-en pressure when you inhale. Re-peated treatments of gradually increasing pressure may be needed for certain trigger points.

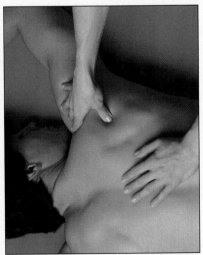

Kneel next to your partner. Use the ball of your thumb to apply pressure to a trigger point. Lean over so that you can use the weight of your upper body for added pressure. Spread your fingers to form a base and place your other hand nearby for support. Maintain the pressure for 10-15 seconds.

LOWER BACK TRIGGER POINT

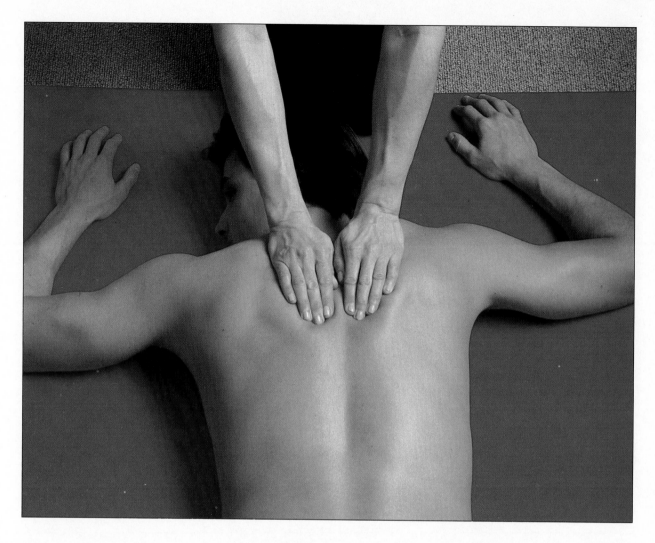

Massage/1

The relaxation that massage induces is more than superficial. A good massage can have such important physiological benefits that massage therapy has gained increased acceptance in recent years as part of muscle rehabilitation programs for some back pain victims.

Massage dilates blood vessels, thereby stimulating circulation. The result is a cleansing process in which waste materials that have collected in the muscles and created pain are flushed out. If you are experiencing acute pain, only a licensed professional should attempt massage.

However, if you are not in pain, you can attain some of the benefits of massage by having a partner perform on you the sequence shown here and on pages 120-123.

To prepare for a massage, lie on a mat in a warm room. Your partner should work deeply into your muscles, but never to the point of causing any pain; also, massage should never put pressure directly on the spine. As the massage progresses, your skin will redden. Called hyperemia, this painless condition is due to the increase in circulation and indicates the overall effectiveness of the massage.

Kneel at your partner's head and place your hands flat on either side of the spine. Stroke firmly straight down the back to the hip bones. Lightly glide your hands back to the neck, keeping your fingertips on the back. Repeat five times.

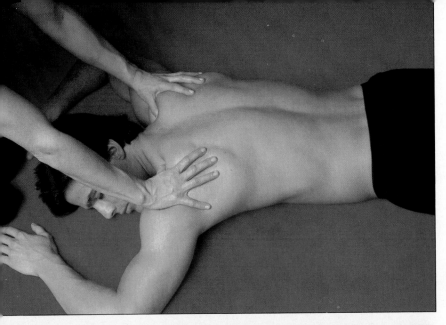

Place your thumbs on either side of the base of your partner's neck and spread your fingers as a base. Stroke outward and back along the top of the shoulders, pressing deeply into the muscle. Repeat five times.

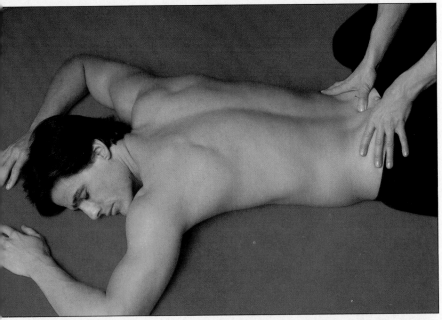

Straddle your partner's legs and place your thumbs on the sacrum, at the base of the spine. Spread your fingers. Rotate your thumbs in small circles, moving around to cover the entire sacrum.

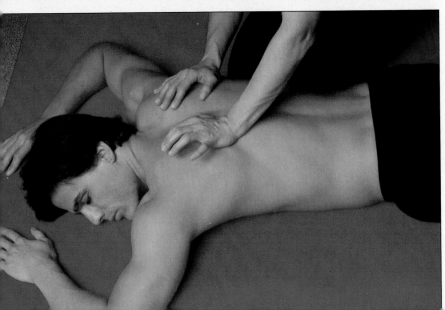

Move to your partner's side. Place one hand on the far side of the spine; rest your other hand on the upper back for support. Starting at the base of the neck, rotate your palm in small circles and push the muscle away from the spine. Work to the top of the buttocks. Perform two repetitions. Then switch arms and work on the side of the back closest to you, this time pulling toward you and away from the spine.

119

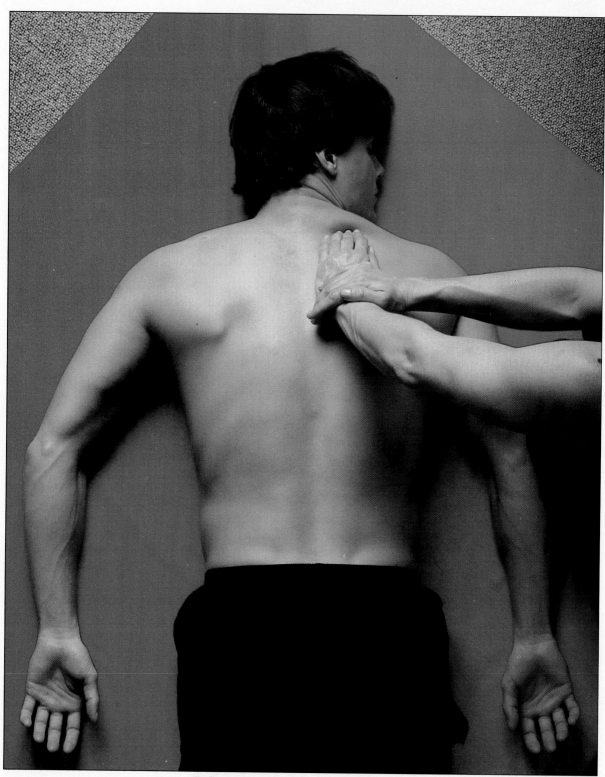

Massage/2

Place one hand on top of the other and make broad circles around the shoulder blade, pressing with your palm. Do not press on the bone itself or on the spine. Repeat five times. Switch shoulders and repeat.

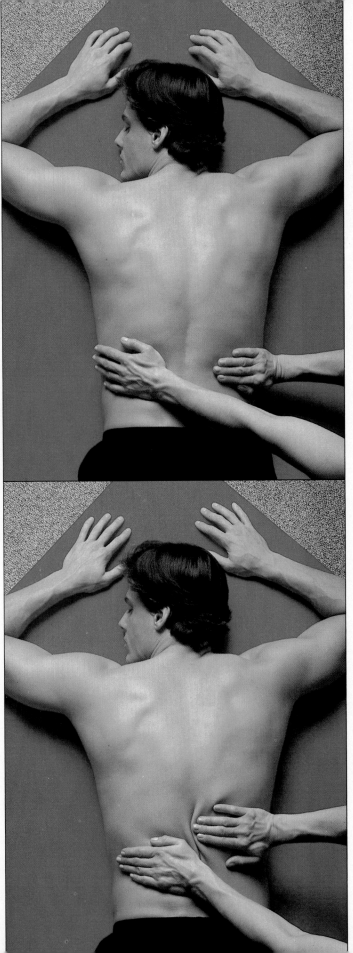

Place your hands on either side of your partner's waist *(left)*. Pressing with your palms, bring your hands toward each other *(bottom)*, avoiding pressure as they cross the spine. Your hands should end in the opposite position from where they started. Repeat this alternating, crossing motion as you work upward to the shoulders, then back down again. Perform two repetitions.

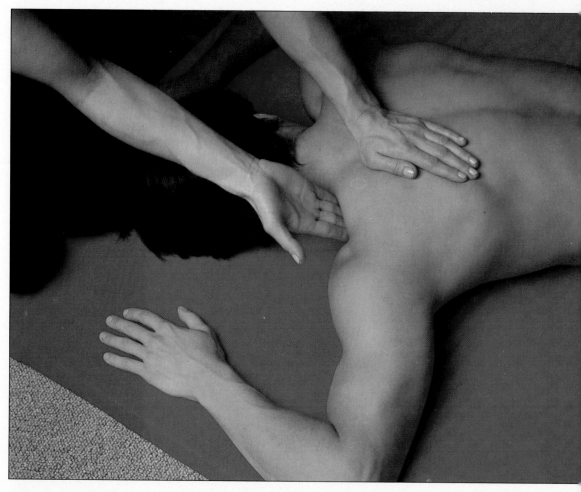

Massage/3

Move back to your partner's head. Put
your left hand on his left shoulder for
support. Place the fingertips of your right
hand beneath your partner's left shoulder.
Stroke along the inside of the shoulder
(above), up the neck to the base of the
skull, twisting your wrist as you work up
the neck *(above right).* Return and repeat
five times, then work up the other side.

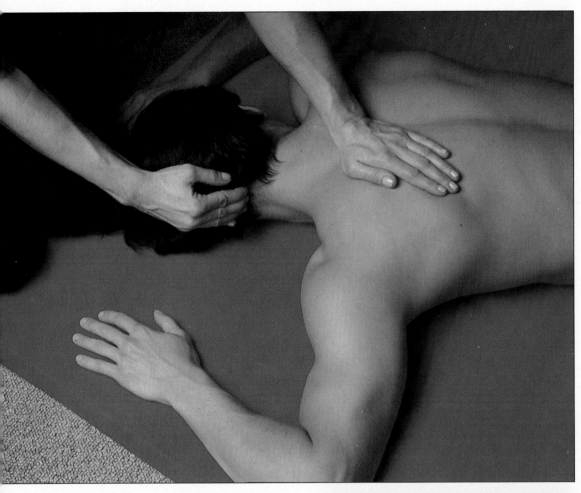

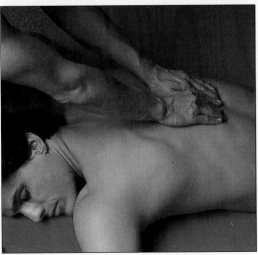

Finish the massage by repeating the first stroke, shown on page 118, down either side of the spine.

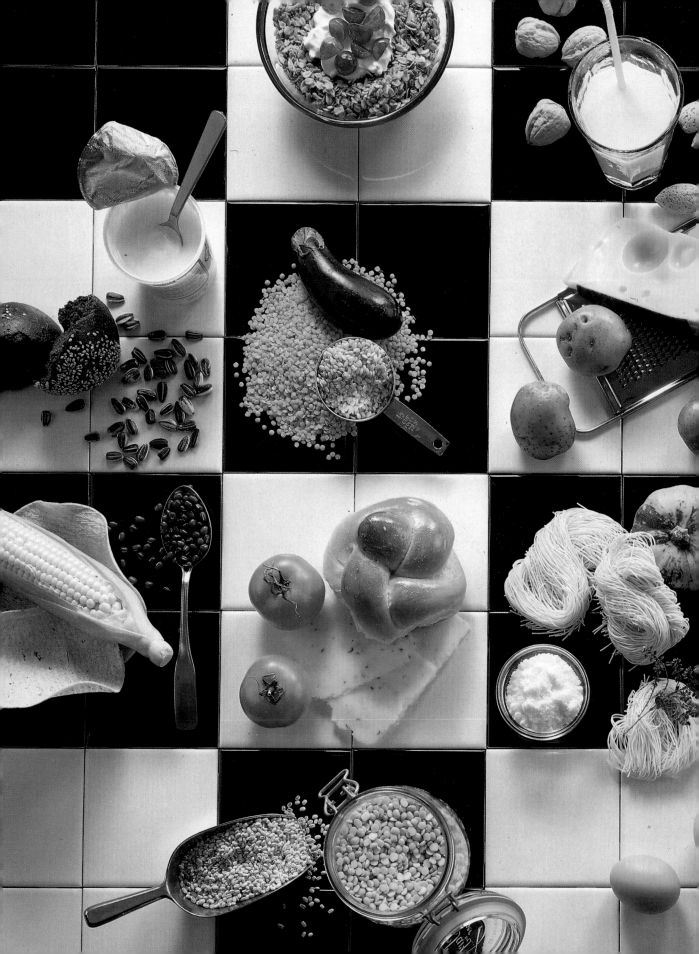

CHAPTER FIVE

Diet and Your Back

The right way to eat to minimize back problems

A lthough being overweight does not condemn you automatically to an aching back, extra pounds can put added stress on your back in several ways. Carrying excessive body fat can result in bad posture, which may make the lower back particularly vulnerable to pain or injury. Studies show that because overweight people exercise less often than people of average weight, their middle-body muscles tend to be less flexible and more flaccid, which tends to put extra stress on the spine. Controlling your weight with diet and exercise is therefore one of the best strategies for avoiding back problems.

The key to an effective weight-control diet is restricting your fat intake. And because red meat is a major source of fat in the diet of most Americans, substituting lowfat meatless recipes for some or all of the meat dishes you usually consume can help you lose weight, maintain a desired weight and reduce your risk of cardiovascular disease. Dishes devoid of red meat, poultry and fish are generally lower in fat — ounce for ounce — than any other type of dish, and thus lower in calories.

A modified vegetarian regimen that includes dairy products and eggs, along with fruit, vegetables, legumes and grains, is called a lacto-ovo vegetarian diet. Such a diet remains low in fat as long as its dairy products are based on skim or lowfat milk, rather than whole milk, and it limits vegetable shortening, oil, butter and lard — which together contribute 44 percent of dietary fat in the American diet — as well as nuts. One recent study comparing 92 lacto-ovo vegetarians and 113 meat eaters found that the vegetarians weighed 16 pounds less than the meat eaters, on average, when such factors as height and body structure were taken into account. Part of this weight advantage may also be due to a difference in lifestyle, since people who choose to be lacto-ovo vegetarians tend to be more active and more diet-conscious than most meat eaters.

In addition to reducing calorie intake, cutting out red meat can lower serum cholesterol levels. A survey of 116 men and women indicated that the vegetarians had blood cholesterol levels averaging 33 percent lower than the nonvegetarians. To maintain a level of blood cholesterol that minimizes your risk of heart attacks and strokes, you should restrict your consumption of egg yolks as well as red meat. One yolk contains approximately 300 milligrams of cholesterol, the amount the American Heart Association recommends as the daily maximum for an adult.

Lacto-ovo vegetarians eating a varied and balanced diet do not need to worry about nutritional deficiencies of calcium and vitamin B_{12}, which are sometimes lacking in the diet of pure vegetarians. However, getting enough iron on a lacto-ovo vegetarian diet can be a problem. Eating vegetables such as spinach, Swiss chard and beet greens, which contain iron, can help. If you cut back or eliminate meat from your diet, you will find that some of the best lowfat protein substitutes are legumes, which include peanuts and the mature or dried seeds of pod-bearing plants, such as lentils, split peas and kidney beans. Like most other plant-derived foods, legumes contain unsaturated fat, which is associated with reducing elevated blood cholesterol levels. Saturated fats, found chiefly in animal products like meat, eggs and milk fat, are associated with high blood pressure, diabetes and the elevated cholesterol levels that are implicated in heart disease.

Legumes by themselves are abundant sources of many vitamins and minerals, but except for soybeans, they are not complete protein since they lack one of the nine essential amino acids, the basic units of protein that cannot be synthesized by the body and must be obtained from food. Combining legumes with any grain or seed or a small amount of animal protein can provide the complete protein that the body needs to build and maintain muscles, organs and antibodies. For example, in the Lentil Tabbouleh in Pita Pockets on page 132, combining lentils with bulgur provides complete protein. Foods that

The Basic Guidelines

For a moderately active adult, the National Institutes of Health recommends a diet that is low in fat, high in carbohydrates and moderate in protein. The institutes' guidelines suggest that no more than 30 percent of your calories come from fat, that 55 to 60 percent come from carbohydrates and that no more than 15 percent come from protein. A gram of fat equals nine calories, while a gram of protein or carbohydrate equals four calories; therefore, if you eat 2,100 calories a day, you should consume approximately 60 grams of fat, 315 grams of carbohydrate and no more than 75 grams of protein daily. If you follow a lowfat/high-carbohydrate diet, your chance of developing heart disease, cancer and other life-threatening diseases may be considerably reduced.

◆ The nutrition charts that accompany each of the lowfat/high-carbohydrate recipes in this book include the number of calories per serving, the number of grams of fat, carbohydrate and protein in a serving, and the percentage of calories derived from each of these nutrients. In addition, the charts provide the amount of calcium, iron and sodium per serving.

◆ Calcium deficiency may be associated with periodontal disease — which attacks the mouth's bones and tissues, including the gums — in both men and women, and with osteoporosis, or bone shrinking and weakening, in the elderly. The deficiency may also contribute to high blood pressure. The recommended daily allowance for calcium is 800 milligrams a day for men and women. Pregnant and lactating women are advised to consume 1,200 milligrams daily; a National Institutes of Health consensus panel recommends that postmenopausal women consume 1,200 to 1,500 milligrams of calcium daily.

◆ Although one way you can reduce your fat intake is to cut your consumption of red meat, you should make sure that you get your necessary iron from other sources. The Food and Nutrition Board of the National Academy of Sciences suggests a minimum of 10 milligrams of iron per day for men and 18 milligrams for women between the ages of 11 and 50.

◆ High sodium intake is associated with high blood pressure. Most adults should restrict sodium intake to between 2,000 and 2,500 milligrams a day, according to the National Academy of Sciences. One way to keep sodium consumption in check is not to add table salt to food.

combine to provide all the essential amino acids are called complementary proteins. The Peach Muffins on page 130, in which grains from the cereal and flour are complemented by the eggs and milk, and the Blue Cheese Spread with Tortilla Triangles on page 141, in which corn tortillas combine with cheese, provide complete protein.

The lacto-ovo vegetarian dishes in this chapter can form the basis of a low-calorie eating plan that may help you control or lower your weight and thereby help safeguard your back. Carbohydrates and protein contribute more than 80 percent of the calories in the recipes, while fat accounts for less than 20 percent. Besides being low in fat and mostly cholesterol-free, such dishes confer several other nutritional advantages. They are high in fiber, the edible but indigestible part of plants that aids in digestion and other bodily functions and that may contribute to weight control; and they contain all the important vitamins and minerals.

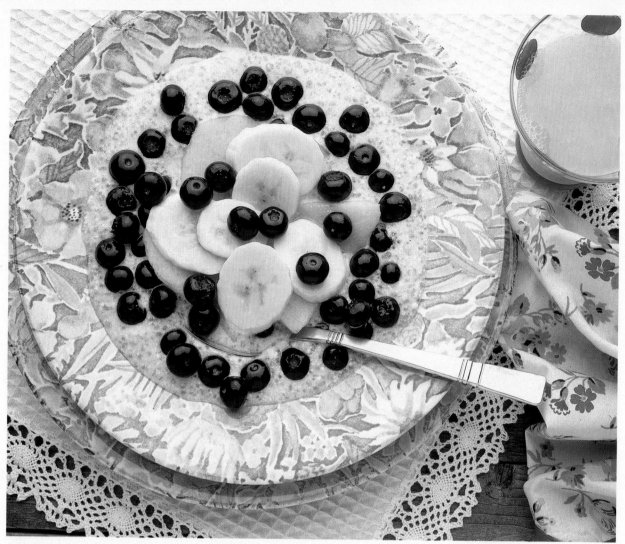

Fruited Ricotta Tapioca

Breakfast

FRUITED RICOTTA TAPIOCA

A pleasant change from cereal, this fruit-topped breakfast pudding is a good lowfat source of calcium, potassium and vitamins A and C.

CALORIES per serving	285
70% Carbohydrates	51 g
13% Protein	10 g
17% Fat	6 g
CALCIUM	191 mg
IRON	1 mg
SODIUM	116 mg

10 tablespoons frozen
   apple juice concentrate
1/4 cup quick-cooking tapioca
1 cup part skim-milk
   ricotta cheese

2 large egg whites
1 tablespoon brown sugar
1 medium-size mango
1 banana
1 cup fresh or frozen blueberries

Stir together the apple juice concentrate, tapioca and 1 cup of water in a small saucepan and set aside for 5 minutes. Bring the mixture to a boil over medium-low heat, stirring occasionally, and cook for 1 minute; remove the pan from the heat and set aside for 30 minutes, or until cool to the touch. Meanwhile, in a medium-size bowl whisk together the ricotta, egg whites and sugar until smooth. Fold the ricotta mixture into the cooled tapioca and spoon the mixture into 4 individual dessert dishes. Cover the dishes with plastic wrap and refrigerate for at least 4 hours, or overnight.

Just before serving, pit the mango and cut it into 1/2-inch-thick slices. Peel the banana and cut it into 1/4-inch-thick slices. Garnish each serving of tapioca with mango and banana slices and blueberries. **Makes 4 servings**

RASPBERRY-RICE SHAKE

This meal-in-a-glass gives you about the same amount of protein as two strips of bacon and two eggs, but it has only one fifth the fat. This shake also supplies 10 grams of fiber, while bacon and eggs have none.

1/2 cup cooked brown rice	3/4 cup plain lowfat yogurt
1 banana, peeled	1/4 cup skim milk
1 cup frozen raspberries	2 teaspoons honey

CALORIES per serving	453
78% Carbohydrates	92 g
13% Protein	16 g
9% Fat	5 g
CALCIUM	433 mg
IRON	2 mg
SODIUM	153 mg

Place the rice in a food processor or blender and process until puréed, scraping down the sides of the container with a rubber spatula. Add the banana and process for another 30 seconds, or until the mixture is as smooth as possible. Add the raspberries, yogurt, milk and honey, and process for another 15 seconds, or until blended. Serve immediately. **Makes 1 serving**

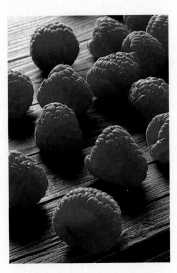

SKILLET RICE PANCAKE

Many people eat high-fat fast-food breakfasts for the sake of convenience, but this dense, crusty rice cake, which will keep for up to three days in the refrigerator, is just as convenient and much lower in fat.

2 cups cooked white rice (2/3 cup raw)	1/4 teaspoon ground cinnamon
2 large eggs plus 1 egg white	1/4 teaspoon vanilla extract
2 tablespoons honey	1/4 teaspoon grated lemon peel
1 Granny Smith apple	2 teaspoons vegetable oil

In a medium-size bowl stir together the rice, eggs and honey; set aside. Wash and core but do not peel the apple, then grate it into a small bowl and squeeze it dry. Add the apple, cinnamon, vanilla and lemon peel to the rice mixture and stir to combine.

Heat 1 teaspoon of oil in a medium-size nonstick skillet over medium heat. Add the rice mixture and pat it into an even layer. Cover the skillet and cook for 5 minutes, or until the bottom of the pancake is golden and the top is dry. To turn over the pancake, slide it onto a plate, cover with another plate and invert. Heat the remaining oil in the skillet. Slide the pancake into the skillet cooked side up and reduce the heat to low. Cook the pancake, uncovered, for about 5 minutes, or until golden and cooked through. Cut into quarters and serve warm, or cool the pancake slightly, then refrigerate it and serve cold.

Makes 4 servings

CALORIES per serving	229
69% Carbohydrates	39 g
10% Protein	6 g
21% Fat	5 g
CALCIUM	30 mg
IRON	2 mg
SODIUM	48 mg

PEACH MUFFINS

Although made with little fat, these muffins are so moist they can be eaten without butter or jam, which could add 50 to 100 calories.

CALORIES per muffin	140
70% Carbohydrates	26 g
10% Protein	4 g
20% Fat	3 g
CALCIUM	50 mg
IRON	2 mg
SODIUM	153 mg

1 cup whole-bran cereal
1 1/4 cups unbleached
  all-purpose flour
1/2 cup whole-wheat flour
1 teaspoon baking powder
1 teaspoon baking soda
1/4 teaspoon ground cinnamon

1 1/2 cups buttermilk
3 tablespoons vegetable oil
1/4 cup honey
2 large eggs, lightly beaten
1 1/2 cups dried peaches
  (9 ounces), coarsely diced

Preheat the oven to 375° F. Line 18 muffin tin cups with paper liners.

In a large bowl stir together the cereal, all-purpose flour, whole-wheat flour, baking powder, baking soda and cinnamon, and make a well in the center. In a medium-size bowl beat together the buttermilk, oil, honey and eggs. Pour the buttermilk mixture into the dry ingredients, add the peaches and stir just to combine. Divide the batter among the muffin tin cups and bake for 20 to 25 minutes, or until the muffins are lightly browned.   Makes 18 muffins

BLUEBERRY-ORANGE MILKSHAKE

Skim milk and fruit make this a good lowfat source of the minerals calcium and potassium.

CALORIES per serving	106
77% Carbohydrates	21 g
18% Protein	5 g
5% Fat	1 g
CALCIUM	190 mg
IRON	.2 mg
SODIUM	64 mg

1 navel orange
2/3 cup frozen blueberries

1 cup skim milk

Grate 2 teaspoons of peel from the orange, being careful not to include any of the white pith; set aside. Peel and segment the orange; remove and discard the membranes. Place the segments in a plastic bag and freeze them for 3 to 4 hours, or until frozen solid.

Place the blueberries, the orange sections and peel in a food processor or blender and process until puréed, scraping down the sides of the container with a rubber spatula. Add the milk and process for 1 minute, or until well blended. Pour the shake into 2 tall glasses and serve.   Makes 2 servings

QUICK BROWN RICE PUDDING

Instead of cereal and milk, try this breakfast "pudding": It is a better source of protein and fiber than most packaged cereals. You can cook rice especially for this recipe, or use leftover rice.

CALORIES per serving	203
82% Carbohydrates	42 g
11% Protein	6 g
7% Fat	2 g
CALCIUM	158 mg
IRON	2 mg
SODIUM	46 mg

1/2 cup plain lowfat yogurt
1 1/2 teaspoons molasses
1 teaspoon honey
1/2 teaspoon vanilla extract

1 cup cooked brown rice
  (1/3 cup raw)
2 tablespoons dried currants

In a small bowl stir together the yogurt, molasses, honey and vanilla. Stir in the rice and currants. Chill before serving, if desired.   Makes 2 servings

Lunch

HERBED POTATOES AU GRATIN

Potatoes baked with cheese can be loaded with fat, but this version gets its flavor from herbs and onions, and uses just 2 tablespoons of cheese.

1 1/2 pounds new potatoes

1 tablespoon butter, melted

1 tablespoon unbleached
   all-purpose flour

1/4 cup chopped fresh parsley

1 1/2 teaspoons fresh rosemary

1 teaspoon minced garlic

1/4 teaspoon black pepper

1 1/2 cups skim milk

3/4 cup sliced onions

2 tablespoons grated
   Swiss cheese

CALORIES per serving	225
69% Carbohydrates	39 g
14% Protein	8 g
17% Fat	4 g
CALCIUM	171 mg
IRON	2 mg
SODIUM	130 mg

Preheat the oven to 375° F. Slice the unpeeled potatoes 1/4 inch thick and place them in a bowl of cold water. Melt the butter in a small saucepan over medium-low heat. Stir in the flour, half the parsley, the rosemary, garlic and pepper. Gradually add the milk, stirring until thick and smooth; set aside.

Drain and dry the potatoes; place half in a 9-inch round baking dish. Top with half the onions, then layer in the remaining potatoes and onions. Pour on the sauce, cover the dish with foil and bake for 30 minutes. Stir the potatoes gently and bake for another 30 minutes. Stir again, sprinkle the cheese on top and bake, uncovered, for 10 to 15 minutes more, or until the cheese is golden brown. Sprinkle with the remaining parsley and serve.   Makes 4 servings

Herbed Potatoes au Gratin

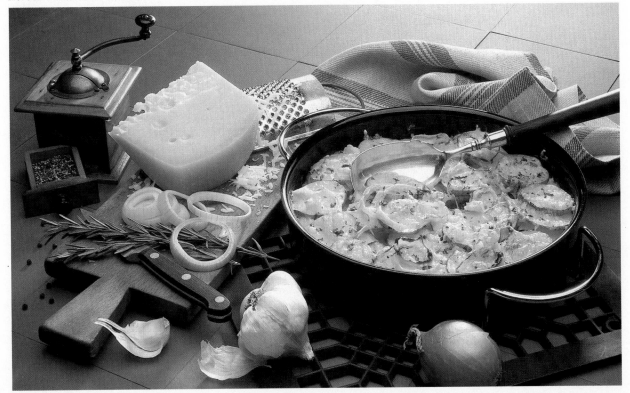

VEGETABLE-BRIE MELT

CALORIES per serving	208
65% Carbohydrates	34 g
15% Protein	8 g
20% Fat	5 g
CALCIUM	80 mg
IRON	3 mg
SODIUM	506 mg

Creamy-tasting Brie gives this sandwich a rich taste, but the topping consists mainly of vegetables, with less than half an ounce of cheese per serving.

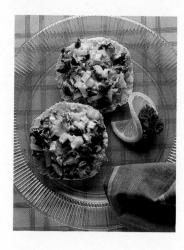

1 1/2 cups shredded spinach
1 cup shredded carrots
2/3 cup coarsely
   chopped mushrooms
1/3 cup coarsely
   chopped shallots

1 1/2 ounces Brie, chilled and
   finely diced (1/4 cup)
1/4 cup plain lowfat yogurt
1 tablespoon Dijon-style mustard
1/4 teaspoon black pepper
4 English muffins

Preheat the oven to 375° F. In a medium-size bowl combine the spinach, carrots, mushrooms, shallots, Brie, yogurt, mustard and pepper, and stir with a wooden spoon until well blended; set aside. Split and toast the muffins, and place them cut side up on a baking sheet. Spoon about 1/3 cup of the vegetable mixture on each muffin half and bake for 10 minutes, or until heated through. Divide the muffins among 4 plates and serve.   Makes 4 servings

LENTIL TABBOULEH IN PITA POCKETS

The combination of lentils, a legume, and bulgur, a whole grain, makes these sandwiches an excellent lowfat source of protein and iron.

1 cup lentils
1 cup diced onion
2 garlic cloves, minced
3/4 cup bulgur
1 cup finely chopped
   fresh parsley
1 cup finely chopped fresh mint
1 1/2 teaspoons dried thyme
1 1/2 teaspoons dried oregano

Hot pepper sauce
1 tablespoon vegetable oil
1 teaspoon grated lemon peel
Eight 1-ounce pita breads
1 small cucumber
2 ounces feta cheese,
   rinsed and drained
8 large Romaine lettuce leaves,
   torn into bite-size pieces

CALORIES per serving	278
71% Carbohydrates	50 g
16% Protein	12 g
13% Fat	4 g
CALCIUM	103 mg
IRON	5 mg
SODIUM	276 mg

Place the lentils, onion, garlic and 3 cups of water in a medium-size saucepan and cook over medium heat for 30 minutes, or until the lentils are tender. Stir in the bulgur, then add half the parsley and mint, and cook over low heat for 2 minutes. Add the thyme, oregano, and pepper sauce to taste, then cover the pan, remove it from the heat and set it aside to cool to room temperature. (If the pan is not kept covered, the bulgur will not absorb the liquid properly.)

When the lentil mixture is cool, pour off any excess liquid, pressing the mixture gently with a slotted spoon. (It should be firm enough to retain the impression of the spoon.) Transfer the mixture to a bowl and stir in the remaining mint and parsley, the oil and lemon peel. Cover the bowl and refrigerate the mixture for at least 2 hours, or until well chilled.

Just before serving, wrap the pita breads in foil and warm them in a 200° F oven. Meanwhile, peel, seed and thinly slice the cucumber and finely dice the feta cheese. Cut open one end of each pita bread. Place some Romaine in each pita. Divide the lentil mixture equally among the sandwiches and top with some of the feta and cucumber.

Makes 8 servings

CREAM OF TOMATO SOUP WITH CROUTONS

This soup has the same amount of protein — but one sixth the fat and half the sodium — of canned tomato soup prepared with whole milk.

CALORIES per serving	**124**
78% Carbohydrates	26 g
16% Protein	5 g
6% Fat	1 g
CALCIUM	112 mg
IRON	2 mg
SODIUM	441 mg

One 14-ounce can plum tomatoes
1 cup tomato juice
1/2 pound new potatoes, peeled and diced
1 1/4 cups diced red bell peppers
1 cup coarsely chopped onion

3 tablespoons chopped fresh coriander
1 garlic clove, crushed and peeled
1/4 teaspoon pepper
1 slice whole-wheat bread
3/4 cup skim milk

Preheat the oven to 375° F. In a medium-size saucepan combine the tomatoes and their liquid, the tomato juice, potatoes, bell peppers, onion, 2 tablespoons of coriander, the garlic and pepper, and bring to a boil over medium heat. Cover the pan, reduce the heat to low and simmer for 15 minutes. Meanwhile, cut the bread into 1/2-inch cubes, spread them on a baking sheet and bake for 5 to 10 minutes, or until golden; set aside to cool.

Remove the pan of soup from the heat and set aside to cool for a few minutes. Purée the soup in a food processor or blender for 1 minute, or until smooth. With the machine running, gradually add the milk. Return the soup to the pan and reheat it over medium-high heat. Ladle the soup into 4 bowls, top it with croutons and garnish with the reserved coriander. Makes 4 servings

ASPARAGUS FRITTATA

Plenty of vegetables, very little oil and less than one egg per serving make this Italian-style omelet a filling and nutritious lunch.

CALORIES per serving	**321**
63% Carbohydrates	51 g
18% Protein	15 g
19% Fat	7 g
CALCIUM	120 mg
IRON	4 mg
SODIUM	522 mg

2 teaspoons olive oil
2 cups diced red bell peppers
1 cup thinly sliced leeks
1/2 cup chopped red onion
2 garlic cloves, minced
3 cups blanched 1-inch asparagus pieces
1 cup sliced mushrooms
1/2 pound unpeeled new potatoes, boiled and sliced (2 cups)

4 fresh plum tomatoes, peeled, seeded and chopped
4 large eggs
1/2 cup lowfat milk (1%)
2 tablespoons grated Parmesan
1/4 cup chopped fresh parsley
1/2 teaspoon dried tarragon
1/2 teaspoon salt
1/4 teaspoon pepper
3/4 pound loaf Italian bread

Heat the oil in a large, flameproof, nonstick skillet over medium heat. Add the bell peppers, leeks, onion and garlic, and sauté for 5 minutes. Add the asparagus and mushrooms, and cook for 4 minutes. Stir in the potatoes and tomatoes, and cook, stirring occasionally, for 3 minutes. Meanwhile, in a medium-size bowl whisk the eggs, milk, Parmesan, parsley, tarragon, salt and pepper. Pour the mixture into the skillet, lifting the vegetables so that the eggs can flow underneath. Increase the heat to medium-high and cook for 10 minutes, or until the eggs are almost set. Meanwhile, preheat the broiler. Broil the frittata 6 inches from the heat for 1 minute, or until the top is lightly browned. Meanwhile, slice the bread. Carefully invert the frittata onto a platter, cut it into 6 wedges and serve it with the bread. Makes 6 servings

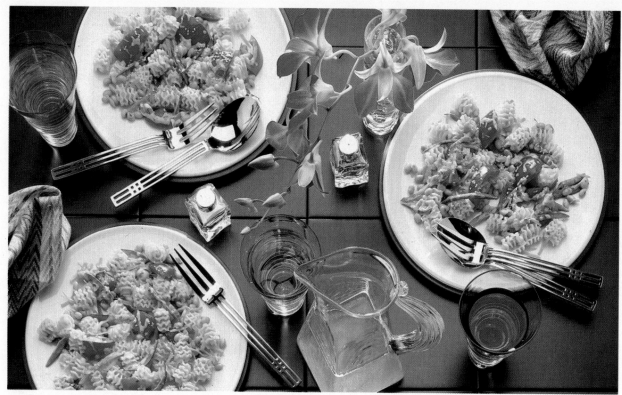

Double-Soy Pasta Salad

Dinner
....

DOUBLE-SOY PASTA SALAD

Soybeans are among the best nonmeat protein sources. Miso, a Japanese flavoring paste, is made from fermented soybeans.

CALORIES per serving	326
71% Carbohydrates	59 g
18% Protein	15 g
11% Fat	4 g
CALCIUM	107 mg
IRON	5 mg
SODIUM	155 mg

1/4 cup dried soybeans, soaked
  overnight in cold water
1 pound tomatoes
1/4 pound carrots
1/4 pound snow peas
1/2 pound pasta ruffles
  or spirals

1 tablespoon plus 1 teaspoon
  light miso
1/4 teaspoon ground ginger
1/4 teaspoon black pepper
1/4 cup plain lowfat yogurt
1 tablespoon chopped parsley
1 teaspoon toasted sesame seeds

Drain the soybeans, add fresh cold water to cover them and bring them to a boil over medium heat. Cover the pan, reduce the heat to low and simmer for 1 hour, or until the soybeans are just tender. Skim off and discard the skins, which will float to the surface. While the soybeans are cooking, core the tomatoes and cut them into chunks. Trim, peel and grate the carrots. Trim the snow peas. Bring a medium-size saucepan of water to a boil and blanch the snow peas for 30 seconds, or until they turn bright green; rinse them under cold running water and set them aside to drain.

    Drain the soybeans and set them aside to cool. Bring a large pot of water to a boil. Cook the pasta for 10 minutes, or according to the package directions, until al dente. Meanwhile, for the dressing stir together the miso, ginger and pepper in a small bowl. Gradually stir in the yogurt, then add 1/4 cup of cold water and stir until smoothly blended; set aside. Cut the snow peas into slivers. When the pasta is done, drain it, rinse it under cold water and set it aside to drain thoroughly.

To serve, place the pasta, tomatoes, carrots, snow peas and soybeans in a large bowl. Pour on the dressing, sprinkle the salad with parsley and sesame seeds, and toss gently to combine.   Makes 4 servings

BEAN-STUFFED PARATHAS

These Indian griddle breads are low in fat because the dough contains less shortening than usual. The spicy filling is very high in protein.

CALORIES per serving	426
69% Carbohydrates	76 g
16% Protein	17 g
15% Fat	7 g
CALCIUM	70 mg
IRON	5 mg
SODIUM	294 mg

1/4 cup dried chickpeas
1/2 cup yellow lentils
1/2 cup chopped onion
1 low-sodium vegetable
 bouillon cube
2 tablespoons minced fresh ginger
1 1/2 tablespoons low-sodium
 tomato paste

1 tablespoon vinegar
2 teaspoons honey
1 teaspoon ground cumin
1/3 teaspoon red pepper flakes
1/2 teaspoon salt
1 cup whole-wheat flour
1 cup bread flour, approximately
1 1/2 tablespoons olive oil

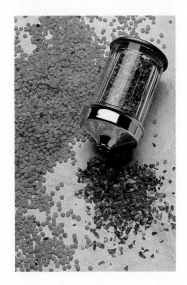

Bring the chickpeas and 2 cups of water to a simmer in a medium-size saucepan, and cook for 2 minutes. Cover the pan and refrigerate overnight.

Bring the chickpeas to a boil over medium heat, cover and cook for 15 minutes. Add the lentils, onion and bouillon cube, and simmer for 45 minutes. Reduce the heat to low, add the ginger, tomato paste, vinegar, honey, cumin, pepper and 1/4 teaspoon salt, and cook, uncovered, stirring occasionally, for 10 minutes. Remove the pan from the heat and set aside to cool.

For the dough, place the whole-wheat flour, 1 cup of bread flour, 1 tablespoon of oil and the remaining salt in a food processor. With the machine running, add 1/2 cup plus 2 tablespoons of water and process for 45 seconds, or until a smooth, elastic dough is formed. Place the dough in a plastic bag, close the top and set aside to rest in a warm place for about 30 minutes.

Lightly flour the work surface and roll out the dough into a 15-inch disk. Brush the dough with the remaining oil, then roll it into a log. With the rolling pin, flatten the log slightly, sealing the ends. Cut the log crosswise into 12 equal pieces. Place one piece of dough on the work surface and roll it out to a 5-inch disk. Place a scant 2 tablespoons of filling on the circle of dough, bring the edges together in the center and pinch them to seal the paratha. Turn it over and flatten it to a 4-inch disk. Repeat with the remaining dough, placing the parathas on a sheet of waxed paper.

Heat a medium-size nonstick skillet over medium heat. Place 3 parathas at a time, seam side down, in the skillet and cook for 5 minutes, then turn them and cook for 3 minutes more. Turn them again and cook for another minute. Cook the remaining parathas in the same fashion. Divide the parathas among 4 plates and serve.   Makes 4 servings

Note: You can make the parathas ahead of time and reheat them before serving. Place the parathas on a baking sheet, cover them with foil and heat in a 350° F oven for 10 minutes.

PASTA WITH BELL PEPPER-TOMATO SAUCE

The nutritional benefits of pasta are enhanced by serving it with a lowfat sauce and a modest amount of cheese. With this method of making sauce — simmering all the ingredients together from the start — no oil or butter is needed to sauté the onion and garlic.

CALORIES per serving	285
75% Carbohydrates	54 g
16% Protein	11 g
9% Fat	3 g
CALCIUM	153 mg
IRON	4 mg
SODIUM	292 mg

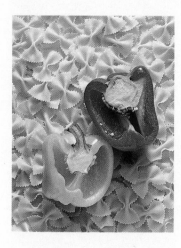

Qne 14-ounce can peeled
  plum tomatoes
1 cup coarsely chopped onion
3 garlic cloves, crushed
  and peeled
1/4 cup chopped fresh basil
1 bay leaf

1/4 teaspoon coarsely ground
  black pepper
Pinch of salt
2 large yellow or red
  bell peppers, slivered
1/2 pound farfalle (bow-tie) pasta
1/4 cup grated Parmesan

For the sauce, combine the tomatoes and their liquid, the onion, garlic, basil, bay leaf, black pepper and salt in a medium-size saucepan, and bring to a boil over medium heat, breaking up the tomatoes with a wooden spoon. Reduce the heat to medium-low and simmer the sauce, uncovered, for 15 minutes.

Add the bell peppers, cover the pan and simmer for 15 minutes more. Meanwhile, bring a large pot of water to a boil. Cook the pasta for 10 minutes, or according to the package directions, until al dente. Drain the pasta and divide it among 4 plates. Remove and discard the bay leaf from the sauce. Spoon the sauce over the pasta, then sprinkle 1 tablespoon of Parmesan over each portion and serve.

Makes 4 servings

POLENTA WEDGES

This version of polenta, an Italian dish made from cooked, cooled cornmeal, is low in fat and high in protein and supplies a good amount of calcium. Serve it with a salad for a satisfying dinner.

CALORIES per serving	277
67% Carbohydrates	47 g
14% Protein	10 g
19% Fat	6 g
CALCIUM	272 mg
IRON	1 mg
SODIUM	255 mg

2 1/2 cups lowfat milk (1%)
3/4 cup yellow cornmeal
2/3 cup golden raisins
2 teaspoons margarine
1/2 teaspoon chopped
  fresh rosemary

1/4 teaspoon salt
Black pepper
Vegetable cooking spray
1/4 cup grated Swiss cheese

Heat the milk in a medium-size heavy-gauge saucepan over medium heat just to the boiling point. Whisk in the cornmeal in a thin, even stream. Reduce the heat to low and simmer, stirring, for about 5 minutes, or until thick. Stir in the raisins, margarine, rosemary, salt, and pepper to taste, and transfer the mixture to a 9-inch pie plate. Let the polenta cool slightly, then cover it loosely with plastic wrap and refrigerate until thoroughly chilled. (The polenta may be made up to 3 days in advance and refrigerated.)

To serve, preheat the oven to 350° F. Cut 4 sheets of foil and spray them with cooking spray. Cut the polenta into quarters, place one piece on each sheet of foil and sprinkle it with grated cheese. Bake for 15 to 20 minutes, or until the polenta is heated through and the cheese is melted and golden.

Makes 4 servings

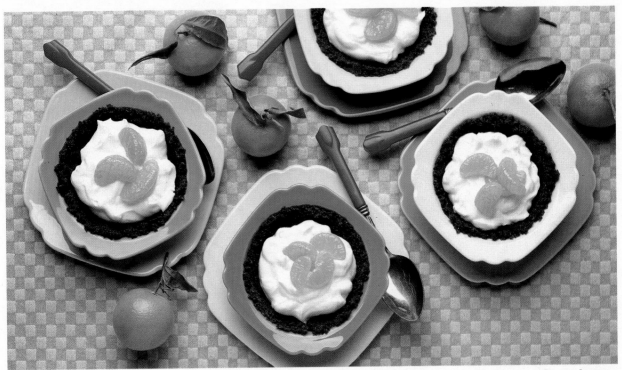

Cheesecake Cups

Dessert

CHEESECAKE CUPS

Cheesecake may derive 60 percent of its calories from fat, with 15 grams per serving. One of these cheesecake cups has only 2 grams.

1 quart plain lowfat yogurt	2 slices pumpernickel bread
3 tablespoons sugar	2 tablespoons honey
1 teaspoon grated lemon peel	1 cup drained juice-packed
1 teaspoon vanilla extract	mandarin orange sections

Line a large strainer with a triple thickness of damp cheesecloth and place it over a medium-size bowl. Gently spoon the yogurt into the strainer, cover it with plastic wrap and place it in the refrigerator for 4 to 6 hours.

Leaving the yogurt in the strainer, stir in the sugar, lemon peel and vanilla, cover and refrigerate for another 4 to 6 hours, or overnight. You should have 1 3/4 to 2 cups of yogurt cheese, depending on the type of yogurt used and the length of time it is drained.

Preheat the oven to 375° F. For the crust, place the bread in the oven and toast it for 10 to 15 minutes, or until it is dry. Place the bread in a food proecessor or blender and process until it is reduced to crumbs. Add the honey and process for another 5 seconds, or until blended. Divide the mixture among 8 dessert dishes or custard cups and press it into the bottom of each dish to form a crust. Spoon a scant 1/4 cup of the yogurt cheese mixture into each cup. Arrange some orange sections on top of each portion and serve.

Makes 8 servings

CALORIES per serving	139
69% Carbohydrates	24 g
19% Protein	7 g
12% Fat	2 g
CALCIUM	218 mg
IRON	4 mg
SODIUM	127 mg

PEACH YOGURT FREEZE

Although commercial frozen yogurts are usually low in fat, they may be loaded with sugar. When you make your own, you can control the sugar content, relying on the natural flavor of fruit for sweetness.

CALORIES per serving	178
75% Carbohydrates	34 g
16% Protein	7 g
9% Fat	2 g
CALCIUM	222 mg
IRON	1 mg
SODIUM	89 mg

One 1-pound can water-packed
 peaches, drained (1 1/2 cups)
1 cup plain lowfat yogurt
1 teaspoon vanilla extract

1 tablespoon brown sugar
2 dried apricot halves, cut into
 thin strips

Place the peaches, yogurt, vanilla and sugar in a food processor or blender and process for 1 minute, or until smooth. Spoon the mixture into 2 dessert dishes and cover with plastic wrap. Freeze the mixture, stirring occasionally to break up the ice crystals, for 2 hours, or until it is frozen but still soft. Just before serving, garnish each portion with apricot strips.   Makes 2 servings

APPLE STRUDEL

While fatty foods produce a sensation of fullness, dietary fiber does the same thing with far fewer calories. Apples and prunes are rich sources of fiber.

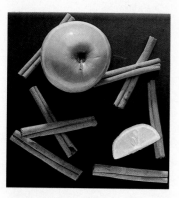

CALORIES per serving	341
77% Carbohydrates	67 g
6% Protein	5 g
17% Fat	7 g
CALCIUM	32 mg
IRON	2 mg
SODIUM	114 mg

1 cup unbleached all-purpose
 flour, approximately
1/4 cup sugar
2 tablespoons margarine,
 well chilled
2 tart apples (about 10 ounces)

1/4 teaspoon lemon juice
10 pitted prunes, chopped
1/4 cup dry bread crumbs
1/4 teaspoon ground cinnamon
1/8 teaspoon ground ginger

In a medium-size bowl stir together 1 cup of flour and 2 tablespoons of sugar. Cut the margarine into small pieces, then using a pastry blender or 2 knives, cut the margarine into the dry ingredients until the mixture is crumbly. Stir in 2 to 3 tablespoons of ice water and mix to form a soft dough. Form the dough into a ball, wrap it in plastic wrap and refrigerate it for at least 30 minutes.

Meanwhile, wash, core and halve but do not peel the apples. Rub one apple half with lemon juice, then wrap and refrigerate it for the garnish. Dice the remaining apples and place them in a medium-size bowl. Add the prunes, bread crumbs, 1 tablespoon of sugar, 1/8 teaspoon of cinnamon and the ginger, and stir until well blended; you should have about 2 cups of filling. Stir together the remaining sugar and cinnamon in a small bowl; set aside.

Preheat the oven to 350° F. Line a baking sheet with foil. Lightly dust the work surface and a rolling pin with flour. Roll the dough out to a 12 x 7-inch rectangle, dusting the surface with additional flour as necessary. Place the filling in the center of the dough to form a 9 x 3-inch rectangle. Bring the long sides of the dough together, fold them over once and pinch them together to seal firmly. Fold in the ends and press firmly to seal them so that the filling does not leak out. Place the strudel seam side down on the baking sheet, sprinkle it with cinnamon-sugar and bake for 25 minutes, or until it is lightly browned at the edges. Let the strudel cool on the baking sheet for 5 minutes. Meanwhile, cut the reserved apple half into 8 slices. Cut the strudel into 4 pieces and garnish each piece with an apple slice.   Makes 4 servings

WHOLE-WHEAT CREPES WITH MIXED FRUIT

These fruit-filled pancakes need no heavy sauce or cream to top them,
and a serving gives you half your daily requirement of vitamin C.

1 cup whole-wheat flour

3 tablespoons sugar

3 large eggs

1 cup frozen unsweetened
  blueberries, thawed and drained

2 oranges, peeled, halved and cut
  crosswise into thin slices

2 tablespoons honey

2 tablespoons lemon juice

1/4 teaspoon ground cardamom

2 kiwi fruit, peeled, halved and
  thinly sliced

1 tablespoon vegetable oil

CALORIES per crêpe	169
67% Carbohydrate	30 g
11% Protein	5 g
22% Fat	4 g
CALCIUM	40 mg
IRON	1 mg
SODIUM	29 mg

For the crêpe batter, place the flour, sugar, eggs and 1 1/2 cups of water in a food processor or blender and process for 1 minute. Transfer the batter to a bowl, cover and refrigerate until needed. (The batter may be made up to 3 hours in advance).

For the filling, combine the blueberries, orange slices, honey, lemon juice and cardamom in a medium-size saucepan and cook over medium heat for 5 minutes, or until the fruit is slightly softened; transfer to a bowl. Drain the kiwi slices, add them to the bowl and toss gently; set aside at room temperature.

Preheat the oven to 200° F. To make the crêpes, stir the batter well to reblend it. Heat a medium-size nonstick skillet over medium-high heat and brush it lightly with oil. Pour in 1/4 cup of batter and swirl the pan to coat the bottom evenly. Cook the crêpe for 1 1/2 minutes, then turn it and cook for another 30 seconds. Transfer the cooked crêpe to a heatproof plate, cover it loosely with foil and place it in the oven to keep warm. Repeat to make a total of 8 crêpes.

To assemble the crêpes, set aside 1/2 cup of filling. Lay each crêpe browned side down on a dessert plate, spoon on about 1/4 cup of filling and fold the sides of the crêpe over it. Top each crêpe with a spoonful of the remaining filling.   Makes 8 servings

Note: The crêpes can be made ahead of time and frozen. To freeze them, interleave them with sheets of wax paper and wrap the stack tightly in foil. To thaw, remove the foil and wax paper, place the crêpes in a baking pan, cover with foil and warm in a 300° F oven for about 10 minutes.

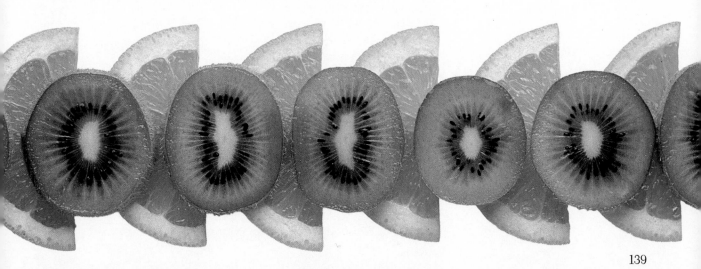

Snacks

· · · · · · · · · · · · ·

STUFFED EGGS

A generous spoonful of spicy potato filling takes the place of the yolks in this version of deviled eggs. The yolks contain all the fat and cholesterol in eggs; almost all the protein is in the whites.

1 pound new potatoes	2 tablespoons dry bread crumbs
8 large eggs	1 tablespoon chopped fresh chives
1 small apple, peeled and cored	1 1/2 teaspoons curry powder
1 large celery stalk	1/4 teaspoon salt
3 tablespoons chutney	Hot pepper sauce
2 tablespoons sour cream	1/4 teaspoon paprika

Place the potatoes and eggs in a medium-size saucepan and add cold water to cover. Bring to a boil over medium heat and cook for 12 minutes. With a slotted spoon, remove the eggs and cool them under cold running water. Cook the potatoes for another 15 minutes, drain and let cool for 15 minutes. Meanwhile, shell the eggs, cut them in half lengthwise and remove and discard the yolks; set aside the whites.

Peel and quarter the potatoes, place them in a medium-size bowl and mash them until smooth. Finely chop the apple and celery in a food processor or by hand, then add them to the mashed potatoes. Add the chutney, sour cream, bread crumbs, 2 teaspoons of chives, the curry powder, salt, and hot pepper sauce to taste and stir until well blended. Spoon the mixture onto the egg whites and place them on a plate; cover with plastic wrap and refrigerate for at least 2 hours. Just before serving, garnish the eggs with the remaining chives and sprinkle them with paprika.   Makes 8 servings

CALORIES per serving	98
72% Carbohydrates	18 g
20% Protein	5 g
8% Fat	1 g
CALCIUM	20 mg
IRON	1 mg
SODIUM	152 mg

Stuffed Eggs

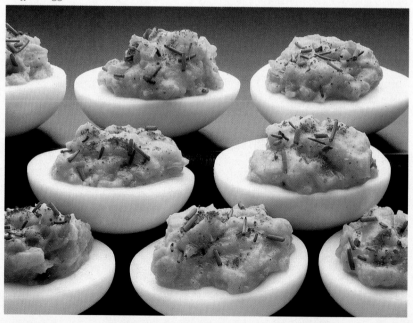

BROWN RICE CRACKERS

Commercial crackers, even "natural" whole-grain varieties, can derive 45 to 50 percent of their calories from saturated fats.

CALORIES per cracker	26
70% Carbohydrates	5 g
11% Protein	1 g
19% Fat	1 g
CALCIUM	4 mg
IRON	.2 mg
SODIUM	74 mg

2 tablespoons skim milk
1 tablespoon walnut oil
1 cup whole-wheat
    flour, approximately

1 cup cooked brown rice
1 teaspoon salt
1/2 teaspoon coarsely ground
    black pepper

In a small bowl stir together the milk, oil and 2 tablespoons of water; set aside. Place 1 cup of flour, the rice, salt and pepper in a food processor and process for 2 to 3 seconds, or just until mixed. With the machine running, add the milk mixture and process just until the dough forms a cohesive mass. If necessary, add up to 1 tablespoon of water. The dough will be sticky but should hold its shape when a small piece is pinched off. Form the dough into a ball, wrap it loosely in plastic wrap and set aside for 15 minutes.

Lightly flour the work surface and a rolling pin. Pat the dough into a disk, then roll it to a 1/2-inch thickness. Let it rest for 10 to 15 minutes, then roll it out again. Repeat the process twice, rolling the dough somewhat thinner each time and dusting with flour if necessary. Let the dough rest between rollings.

Preheat the oven to 350° F. Roll the dough out to a 10 x 9-inch rectangle about 1/8 inch thick. Using a ruler and a sharp knife, cut the dough into thirty 1 x 3-inch rectangles. Place the crackers 1/2 inch apart on a baking sheet and bake for 20 minutes, or until crisp and golden. Transfer the crackers to racks to cool and repeat with the remaining dough. Makes 60 crackers

BLUE CHEESE SPREAD WITH TORTILLA TRIANGLES

The spread is potato-based and the chips are baked, making this a low-fat snack. And, because the complete protein in dairy products complements the incomplete protein in grains, you get more usable protein.

1 pound new potatoes
Four 8-inch corn tortilllas
1/2 cup skim milk
1 ounce blue cheese, crumbled

1 tablespoon chopped
    fresh chives
1/4 teaspoon coarsely ground
    black pepper

Scrub the potatoes, place them in a medium-size saucepan with cold water to cover and bring to a boil over medium heat. Cover the pan, reduce the heat to low and simmer for 20 minutes, or until the potatoes are tender when pierced with a knife. Drain the potatoes and set aside to cool.

Meanwhile, preheat the oven to 500° F. Dip each tortilla in a bowl of water, then cut it into 8 triangles. Place the triangles on a baking sheet and bake for 3 to 4 minutes, or until crisp. Remove the baking sheet from the oven and reduce the oven temperature to 300° F. Return the tortilla triangles to the oven and bake for another 2 to 3 minutes, or until golden brown; set aside.

When the potatoes are cool enough to handle, peel and quarter them. Place them in a medium-size bowl and mash them, then gradually stir in the milk, cheese, chives and pepper. The mixture should be well blended but not completely smooth. Transfer the spread to a serving bowl and serve with the warm tortilla triangles. Makes 4 servings

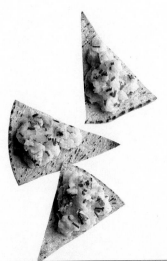

CALORIES per serving	193
71% Carbohydrates	35 g
14% Protein	7 g
15% Fat	3 g
CALCIUM	126 mg
IRON	2 mg
SODIUM	175 mg

PROP CREDITS

Pages 26-29: pants–Gilda Marx Sport, Los Angeles, Calif., pillows and towel–Martex, New York City; page 30: leotard, tights–Dance France LTD, Santa Monica, Calif.; pages 34-39: top, shorts–Athletic Style, New York City, shoes–Nautilus Athletic Footwear, Inc., Greenville, S.C., mat–AMF American, Jefferson, Iowa; pages 36-37: pillow–Martex, New York City; pages 40-55: top–Athletic Style, New York City, shorts–Naturalife, New York City, shoes–Nautilus Athletic Footwear, Inc., Greenville, S.C., mat–AMF American, Jefferson, Iowa; page 43: pillow–Martex, New York City; page 50: pillow–Martex, New York City; page 53: pillow–Martex, New York City; pages 56-67: top, shorts–Athletic Style, New York City, shoes–Nautilus Athletic Footwear, Inc., Greenville, S.C.; page 57: towel–Martex, New York City; pages 58-59: mat–AMF American, Jefferson, Iowa; pages 66-67: chair–Herman Miller, Zeeland, Mich.; page 68: leotard–Marika, San Diego, Calif.; pages 72-93: leotard, tights–Dance France LTD, Santa Monica, Calif.; pages 90-91: towel–Martex, New York City; page 94: sweat pants–Athletic Style, New York City; page 98: kneeling chair–Hag, New York City; lumbar cushion–Leroy Pharmacy, New York City; page 99: lumbar roll, footstool–Leroy Pharmacy, New York City, chair–Herman Miller, Zeeland, Mich.; pages 100-101: shirt, tie, belt, pants–Burberry's LTD, New York City; pages 102-115: shoes–Nautilus Athletic Footwear, Inc., Greenville, S.C.; page 110: vacuum cleaner–Electrolux Corp., New York City; pages 112-113: top–Athletic Style, New York City, futon, sheets, blanket, pillowcases–The Futon Shop, New York City, pillows–Martex, New York City; pages 116-123: shorts–Athletic Style, New York City; mat–AMF American, Jefferson, Iowa; pages 124-125: tiles–Nemo Tile, New York City; page 128: linen placemat–Gear, New York City, spoon–Gorham, Providence, R.I.; page 131: tiles–Nemo Tile, New York City, linen–Frank McIntosh at Henri Bendel, New York City, casserole–Sointu, New York City; page 134: tiles–Nemo Tile, New York City, vase, glasses–Giles and Lewis, New York City, napkins–Gear, New York City, plates–Sointu, New York City, flatware, salt and pepper shakers–Sasaki, New York City, pitcher–Frank McIntosh at Henri Bendel, New York City; page 137: spoons–Mood Indigo, New York City; page 140: tiles–Nemo Tile, New York City.

ACKNOWLEDGMENTS

All cosmetics and grooming products supplied by Clinique Labs, Inc., New York City

Nutrition analysis provided by Hill Nutrition Associates, Fayetteville, N.Y.

Off-camera warm-up equipment: rowing machine supplied by Precor USA, Redmond, Wash.; Tunturi stationary bicycle supplied by Amerec Corp., Bellevue, Wash.

Washing machine and dryer supplied by White-Westinghouse, Columbus, Ohio

Index prepared by Ian Tucker

Production by Giga Communications

PHOTOGRAPHY CREDITS

Exercise photographs by Andrew Eccles; food photographs by Steven Mays, Rebus, Inc.

ILLUSTRATION CREDITS

Page 9, illustration: Dana Burns-Pizer; page 10, illustration: Brian Sisco; page 13, illustration: Dana Burns-Pizer; page 15, illustration: Tammi Colichio; page 16, illustration: Brian Sisco; pages 20-23, illustrations: Kevin Kelly; page 33, illustration: Dana Burns-Pizer; page 71, illustration: Kevin Kelly; pages 103-105, 107, 109, 111, 112-114, illustrations: David Flaherty

Time-Life Books Inc. offers a wide range of fine recordings, including a Rock 'n' Roll Era *series. For subscription information, call 1-800-621-7026, or write TIME-LIFE MUSIC, P. O. Box C-32068; Richmond, Virginia 23261-2068.*

INDEX